PREFACE

In this volume I have endeavored to place before the public a novel method of real scientific massage movements combined with exercises, so that the benefits of both may be obtained simultaneously.

The simplicity of its technic together with its ready personal application make it possible for any individual to achieve excellent results from its use.

The application of scientific massage movements stimulates the nerves, tissues, muscles, organs, vessels, glands and cells much more beneficially and effectively than general exercises. Their combined application is physical culture in its most scientific and perfected form.

In working out a practical presentation of this system, it was noted that the massage movements and the most beneficial exercises could be combined readily and simply (although this must be done in a prescribed way) and that their balanced, logical combination resulted in a method far superior to all other systems of exercises, not only for the maintenance of health, but for special therapeutic and physiologic purposes.

The exercises are chiefly intended for use at home, and will be found to be more advantageous to the individual than any course of physical culture offered anywhere. No gymnastic equipment is necessary and no expenditure, save that of the time required, which will vary mostly from twelve to twenty-five minutes daily according to the time, need and inclination of the individual.

ALBRECHT JENSEN,
New York.

DR. WILLIAM SHARPE
20 West 50th Street,
New York

March,1920.

Mr.Jensen:

DearSir:

Itisapleasur etor ecommendmosthighlyyoursystemofmassage and exercises combined. I have observed the excellent results—from your method of massage alone—in so many of the patients at the Polyclinic Hospital—both in my own patients and in those of the other physicians that I do not hesitate to endorse your statements. The fact that no apparatus is necessary for the combined massage exercises, which are thus automatically graduated according to eachperson'sstr engthandcondition,isamostdesirablefeatur e.

They are especially adapted to be used by men, women and childrenasapermanentphysicalcultur ecourse.

Verytrulyyours,

(Signed)W illiamSharpe.

EDWARD LELAND KELLOGG, M.D.
WILLIAM ALVIN KELLOGG, M.D.
48 West 51st Street
New York

April,1920.

Mr.A.Jensen,
NewYorkCity.

DearSir:

I am glad to have had the privilege of looking over the manuscriptofyoursystemofcombinedmassageandexer cise.

The results so far as I have observed them have been excellent. This combined treatment possesses manifest advantages over either massageorexer cisesgivenseparately .

The fact that no apparatus is needed and that the strength of the individual adapts the course or treatment to his particular need, rendersitgenerallyapplicable.

Verytruly ,

(Signed)E.L.Kellogg.

CONTENTS

SUPPLEMENT

ATHLETIC INSTRUCTORS

The tendency of most instructors or athletes, when presenting exercises, is to lay stress upon the production of large muscles, capable of certain performances. Some even go so far as to relate specific feats, which they are able to accomplish by reason of their great muscular power, which, it may be observed, is not necessarily indicative of good health. Oftentimes they have obtained this muscular strength by other exercises than the ones described in their books, or they have been accustomed to hard work from early youth, or are naturally strong. But the impression is conveyed that any individual can acquire the same muscular strength by practicing their exercises.

It is interesting to note that Sandow in his "Magazine for Physical Culture," criticizes the abdominal muscles of a Danish instructor in athletics by the name of Muller, as almost abnormally developed, and Muller in turn retorts that Sandow's arms and legs are too thick for their length, and his figure is too clumsy. That Mr. Muller has a better figure than Mr. Sandow is true, as is likewise the fact that the latter has given too much attention to heavy-weight lifting. Sandow is not as tall as Muller, however, and quite naturally if a man of small stature has the same muscular development as a taller man, it is conclusive that the figure of the smaller must appear more clumsy.

It does not follow that two persons practicing the same exercises will develop similar figures, although some men and women, who teach or publish courses in physical culture, often give their pupils or readers this impression.

However, any good exercises will improve the figure. What is significant is the fact that Sandow and Muller are arguing so much about a matter of no vital importance. Both might be sound and healthy, even if what they say about each other is true.

In a book of exercises published by Mr. Muller, mention is made of some rubbing or skin exercises, as they are called. These are practically only skin deep, as far as the rubbing is concerned. Mr. Muller correctly admits this in an explanation that the rubbing provides for a kneading of the entire surface of the skin. The English translator of the book likewise explains, in his Introduction, that the rubbing exercises are an endeavor to restore to its due position, the proper care of the skin.

There is a great difference between scientific massage movements and rubbing, although this may not be evident to the layman. While scientific massage movements also benefit the skin, their influence upon the deeper lying vessels, organs, nerves and muscles is of far greater importance.

RESULTANT BAD EFFECTS FROM THE USE OF HEAVY APPARATUS, WEIGHTS AND TOO STRENUOUS EXERCISES

Something similar to what happened to the frog that wanted to be as large as the ox occurs in many a young man, who begins to exercise with heavy apparatus and weights in order to develop his muscles. Usually in the first or second month there will be a marked increase of development of the muscles and believing that this relative development will continue, he becomes over-enthusiastic and works so vigorously that he suffers from his mistake. Then, if the exercises are suddenly stopped and not gradually decreased, and if the poisonous substances and fatigue matter accumulated in the muscles are not removed by massage, the result will be muscles that are too hard and too stiff, with the accompanying ill effects. Such exercises also place too great a strain upon the nerves, heart and other organs of the body. The energy it demands ought to be put to a better purpose; as Jules Claretie of the Theatre Français in Paris aptly said, when discussing some rough sport, "Think though about other things."

Most apparatus used for exercise acts too artificially.

Because a person possesses great muscular strength, it does not necessarily follow that his organs and nerves have a proportionate strength and vitality. Many noteworthy examples of this fallacy may be cited. Thus, for instance, Ellegaard, known as one of the best cycle riders in the world, some fifteen years ago, was rejected as a soldier. John L. Sullivan, the boxer, died of a weak heart. Les Darcy, the boxer from Australia, who was to have fought Jess Willard, succumbed to pneumonia within a few days after his illness, and many other athletic exponents have impaired their health or gone to too early a grave, the victims of professional ambition.

One should be by no means adverse to well developed and strong muscles, so long as the elasticity and rhythm of the movements of the body are unimpaired, but if the nerves and organs have been overtaxed in the development of the muscles, the result is a weaker instead of a stronger individual.

Experiments have shown that while the man with big and hard biceps muscles may be able to lift a heavier weight than the man with more supple and elastic muscles, the latter would lift a smaller weight a greater number of times. Both would improve their performance after five minutes of massage had been applied to the arms.

When practicing the combined massage exercises set forth in this book, the muscles become massaged during each exercise.

The strongest athlete may exert the same strength that he employs in heavy-weight lifting, or apparatus work, when applying these massage movements to the body, without any of the possible ill effects resulting from heavy gymnastic work. The use of such strength in the combined massage exercises will thus result in benefit for the body in the form of massage, and this will greatly assist in re-establishing the vitality that might have been lost by excessive strenuous exercises.

It should not be construed that these arguments are intended as advice to refrain from outdoor exercises and sports. Anyone and everyone should practice and participate in any sports suitable to their temperament, time and purse, but care should be taken not to overtax the strength or vitality.

SPECIAL BENEFIT TO WOMEN FROM THE USE OF THESE EXERCISES

The combined massage exercises are extremely beneficial to women and girls of all ages.

Women suffer more from constipation than men. This may be due to the use of corsets, which at times prevent the respiratory muscles from being put into full play, or hinder the blood from circulating freely and often cause flabbiness or even atrophy to the abdominal and pectoral muscles. It is therefore often the original and chief cause of disorders in the digestive and abdominal organs.

It is especially important that women, looking forward to motherhood, should possess strong and healthy abdominal organs and muscles. These will cause a quick and natural delivery of the child; and children born under such conditions are not likely to suffer deforming injuries, as for instance, the tearing of a nerve leading to an arm (brachial paralysis), etc., which often occurs when artificial means have to be used at their birth.

Pregnancy is, however, not feared so much either for the inconvenience of carrying the infant or its delivery, but chiefly because of the current idea that a woman may lose her girlish appearance or not feel as young as before; this has often happened to many. If from early youth a woman has exercised and trained her abdominal muscles, the state of pregnancy will be less disagreeable. She would also look forward to this state with more hope and delight, if she could be made to realize that by care, massage and exercises of the abdominal muscles, after having recovered from her accouchement, she could regain her former figure and appearance.

The combined massage exercises, Nos. 10, 3, 7 and 5 are most beneficial for the abdominal organs and muscles. The massage movements in Nos. 10 and 3 are especially beneficial, for pelvic exudations; they cause a quicker and more complete removal of same.

If girls of thirteen years of age or younger would begin to practice the combined massage exercises and the breathing exercises for fifteen or twenty minutes each day, irregularities in periodical exudations could be prevented in most cases; the chest would be firmer and it would do much to allow the change into womanhood to proceed without any injury to the nerves or general health.

THE CONSTRUCTION AND CHARACTERISTICS OF THE COMBINED MASSAGE EXERCISES

The chief characteristics of the exercises presented in this book is that scientific or medical massage movements (not mere rubbing) have been combined with the essentials of preliminary gymnastic exercises, such as for instance, bending, stretching and circulating movements of the arms, the bending of the body (trunk) backward, forward and to the side, turning and rolling it to the right or left, and bending and stretching the legs.

By this combined application of the massage movements with the movements of the body, there is also obtained the benefit of the essential characteristics of the Indian Yogis system or concentration exercises, so-called after the old Hindus,—the Yogi. For example, one of their exercises consisted of placing the backs of the hands on the back, and by concentrating the mind on the muscles of the arms a stationary pressure was exerted on that part of the body. Another consisted of clutching the hands firmly (with arms at sides) and rising up on toes, at the same time concentrating the mind on the muscles of the arms and legs. The Yogis also practiced other exercises, in which the hands exerted a stationary pressure on other parts of the body and against a wall.

The few more or less fantastic systems of exercise presented during the last fifty years, which consist mainly in producing an imaginary resistance to the muscles by will power only, originate from the Indian Yogis.

In the exercises presented in this book a natural, better and more agreeable resistance to the muscles of the legs, arms and trunk is secured by stroking and pressing with the hands on the body and limbs. **Here the pressing is not stationary**, as in the Indian and similar exercises, but it is done while the hands are stroking. **This stroking and pressing** is done in such a manner that it is identical with scientific massage movements, some of which have been used by specialists prominent in Europe and America. To the exercises are also added those which in the author's experience at hospitals in New York, have been found to be productive of the best results. The only difference is that they are here joined to the movements of the body and are performed by the individual.

These massage movements have a far greater beneficial effect—therapeutically as well as physiologically—than the body movements themselves, to which they are combined. A brief explanation of their effects may here be interpolated.

1. They bring about increasing activity in the glands and vessels of the skin and muscles. Waste and poisonous substances are carried away by the lymph and blood supply and disposed of through the skin, lungs and kidneys more readily than otherwise.

2. Flabby and atrophied muscles are nourished and restored, while hard and contracted muscles are made more soft and supple; and fatigue matter removed from them.

3. They stimulate and nourish the nerves and through them the tissues and organs of the body.

4. They cause increased combustion in the tissues, more carbonic acid gas is eliminated and more oxygen absorbed, thereby stimulating and increasing respiration through the lungs and skin pores.

5. The massage movements will likewise stimulate and cause increased activity in the digestive organs. The flow of the digestive juices from the liver and pancreas, which are essential for proper digestion and absorption of food, is increased. They assist in preventing engorgement of the liver and are very beneficial to that organ. The stomach and intestines are influenced directly by the mechanical action of the massage movements and indirectly through nourishment of the nerve centres controlling them.

6. The direct action of the kidneys and bladder is also stimulated, so that waste and poisonous substances are eliminated more quickly.

7. The heart is influenced not only by massaging around and over its region, thus stimulating the muscles and nerves surrounding it, but also through the influence of the massage movements on the circulation of the blood. The strength of the heart-beat is thus increased and the number decreased.

8. Weak eyes have been benefited by the effect of massage on the nervous system.

Summarizing, it may be seen that: (1) In the massage exercises the essentials of preliminary gymnasium exercises are included with their resultant benefit. (2) The therapeutic and physiologic beneficial effect of scientific massage movements are obtained. (3) The benefit of the essential characteristics of the concentration system originated by the Hindus is secured and in a much more effective facile and agreeable manner. (4) In addition, there accrue the other general advantages which the massage exercises possess. A few of these may be noted:

a. The maximum of effect with the minimum of effort.

b. The stretching, pressing, stimulating and nourishing of the nerves in a natural way.

c. The avoidance of mental fatigue. The longer the exercises are practiced the more they are liked, because of their agreeable nature and immediate effect.

d. Inasmuch as they are regulated by the pressure of the hands, they may be adapted to any required degree and thus are equally beneficial to all, from the most developed athlete down to the little child old enough to understand their execution.

e. The exercises may also be used in different disordered and diseased conditions of the body, of a mild character, in which massage is helpful. A person with injured legs and even one with no legs at all will be able to practice some of them in a sitting or lying posture; namely, massage exercises Nos. 1, 2, 10 and 12, and without the movements of the body also Nos. 8, 11 and 14.

f. Because they improve the circulation of blood and lymph, enrich the blood, burn away fatty tissues, build up muscles, and have the most beneficial influence on the nerves and glands; they will improve the appearance and the figure of both stout and thin.

g. They will preserve youth and retard old age.

COMMENTARIES AS TO THEIR USE

The massage exercises are chiefly intended to serve as a daily course for men, women and children, in order to preserve and improve their health, vitality, energy and figure.

The best method to adopt is to practice all the combined massage exercises in their order together with a special or general deep breathing exercise at the intervals as explained in Chapter "Synoptic Review," page 78. In this way the massage movements and the movements of the body are applied in the best proportion. Whether the massage exercises are done five, ten or fifteen times each, or more, the time allotted for the deep breathing at the intervals indicated should not exceed fifteen seconds.

Practicing all the exercises from five to fifteen times each in the manner noted will require from twelve to twenty-five minutes (i.e., one performance), which will be most suitable to all who are using them as a daily course. Old and stout persons will probably require a little more time for one performance than is necessary for those who are younger, thinner or more athletic. There is, however, nothing to prevent anyone from increasing the time to half an hour or even longer if desired; or, the performance may be made to last as long as the performer might have been accustomed to exercise in a gymnasium. The average time required for doing each massage exercise five times will be found in the descriptions.

THE PRESSURE OF THE HANDS

The massage exercises not only may be regulated and made more or less vigorous by increasing or decreasing their number and speed, but also by increasing or decreasing the pressure of the hands while stroking the body. They can thus be practiced fifteen times each with a light pressure and not tire as much as if they are practiced five times each with a stronger pressure.

A light pressure is accomplished when practically only the weight of the hands is put into play.

The strongest pressure is exerted when the fingers and hands are used as forcefully as possible.

A moderate pressure is one which is midway between no real pressure and the most forceful.

A strong pressure is then somewhat more forcible than the moderate.

A powerful pressure with the hands will of course give a more effective massage and make the movements of the body and limbs more vigorous, thus influencing the entire body to a greater degree than will a light pressure. However, this does not mean that it is necessary or most practical to utilize the strongest pressure possible, although even that may be done without causing harm, since the massaging of the muscles will automatically prevent any stiffness or ill effects.

It must be remembered that by the strongest pressure is meant the strongest that one is able to exert upon oneself. Let us take, for example, two persons of widely different physical strength, such as a powerful wrestler and a little girl of about ten years of age. If the wrestler uses the strongest pressure possible for him to exert, that pressure would not be harmful to him (provided, of course, that he has had no recent injuries), since his body is proportionately strong. The little girl, however, cannot endure the pressure that the wrestler is able to exert on his body, but she will not be able to press so forcibly. She will, however, be able to endure the strongest pressure that she can exert, because its strength will be in proportion to the strength of her body.

If it is a question as to whether each exercise should be practiced a lesser number of times with the strongest pressure or a greater number of times with a moderate or strong pressure, the latter method is not only advisable but preferable.

Therefore, in most instances a moderate or strong pressure should be used when the same pressure is exerted throughout one performance.

Using different degrees of pressure for one exercise is not only quite practical, but also as effective as using the same pressure for one performance. For instance, if an exercise is practiced five times, the first time a light pressure may be exerted, the second time a moderate, the third time a strong, the fourth also a strong and the fifth a moderate pressure.

If an exercise is done ten times the different degrees of pressure can, of course, be accomplished with more variation. In other words, a changing pressure may be utilized by gradually increasing it each time, until the exercise has been executed five or six times, then gradually decreasing for each of the remaining four or five times. If the exercise is practiced fifteen times, increase the pressure until the seventh or eighth time, decreasing it for each of the remaining times, and so forth.

THE DEGREE OF EXERTION

Whether the massage exercises are practiced a lesser number of times with a strong pressure or a greater number of times with a light pressure and whether they are executed quickly or slowly; each exercise may be practiced until the desired fatigue is induced.

A boxer, wrestler or any other athlete in training may wish to practice the exercises in such a manner and to such an extent that complete fatigue results. The same may be true in the case of stout people who wish to reduce, when the heart and other vital organs are not essentially weakened.

Men, women and children who use the exercises daily for improving and preserving their health will undoubtedly follow a moderate course and do each exercise only until slightly fatigued. However, more strenuous performances may be executed, but care should be taken to avoid all extremes.

If any exercise provokes fatigue, the fifteen seconds deep breathing between that and the next will probably serve to eradicate this. If not, the pause between the massage exercise and the breathing may be prolonged. However, the fatigue feeling resulting from a vigorous or prolonged massage exercise will not last as long as that which results from other exercises with similar exertion. This is due to the influence of the massage movements.

THE BEST TIME FOR THE EXERCISES

While it is well to do exercises in the morning, the majority do not feel inclined to exert themselves vigorously immediately upon arising. Neither is it scientifically correct, since the body has been inactive and in a prone position for several hours. The following procedure is advisable:

Upon arising, practice the general and special breathing exercises without strain, about two times each. This will benefit the heart action and the circulation. Subsequently, or after the bath, practice all the massage exercises from five to ten times each. If there is no time for all, practice exercises No. 7 or 5, or both.

Get the habit of proper breathing from early morning.

If a bath is taken every morning, a warm shower gradually getting cooler is preferable.

The afternoon or evening, about half an hour before dinner, is also a desirable time for exercising, since the flow of the gastric juices will be stimulated and cause the entire digestive system to be in its best condition for the reception of food. It is best not to do any violent exercising within at least three-quarters of an hour after a substantial meal has been taken.

If the massage exercises are practiced for about ten minutes without too much exertion, just before going to bed, it will prove beneficial to sleep.

Before and after a bath in the ocean is also an opportune time for doing the exercises.

It is not intended to convey the impression that all the combined massage exercises must necessarily be performed three times every day, although this might be very good under proper circumstances. They should be done, however, at least once a day, although adherence to this rule may not be feasible at all times. For instance, on a very hot day, with a high degree of humidity, when continual perspiration is induced, it may seem desirable to omit them. However, if only one or two massage exercises are done in the morning it is advisable that all of them, with the breathing exercise, at the intervals, be practiced at least five times each later in the day. Ten times each would be better.

In addition, the special and general deep breathing exercises should be practiced separately for about five minutes once or twice daily.

SPECIAL REMARKS

Each exercise should be done in one uniform rhythmical movement.

The room should be aired, the window open, if this is possible without incurring draught or without too great a drop in the temperature.

One is not likely to take cold when exercising but it is well to dress quickly upon completion of the movements. Of course in the winter the room may be warmed.

If the skin is moist, a bath should be taken or the body wiped with a wet, cool towel and thoroughly dried before the exercises are commenced. If the body and the palms of the hands become moist while exercising, some talcum powder should be sprinkled on the skin.

THE ILLUSTRATIONS

To those, who have read the preceding chapters, it will hardly be necessary to point out, that the exercises demonstrated by a woman are not intended for women only but also for men and children; and likewise the exercises demonstrated by a man—the author—are equally beneficial for women and children.

GENERAL AND DETAILED DESCRIPTION OF THE COMBINED MASSAGE EXERCISES WITH THEIR ANALYSIS AND EFFECTS

(*See also* Synoptic Review)

Exercise No. 1

Massaging with both hands simultaneously from the forehead or each temple up over the top and side of the head and continuing down the back of the head, neck and cervical vertebrae, and thence around both sides of the neck and down each side of the throat; at the same time bending the head forward and backward.

Detailed Description

Position.—Standing or sitting erect in a chair or bed.

EXERCISE No. 1.

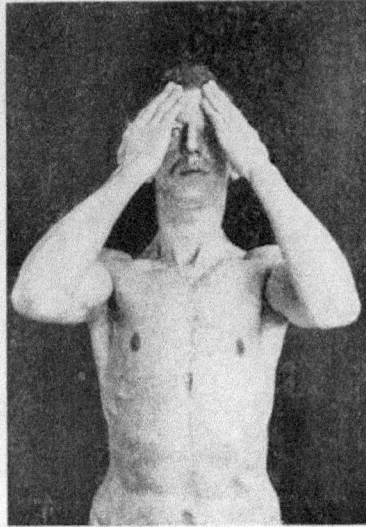

Fig. 1 A.

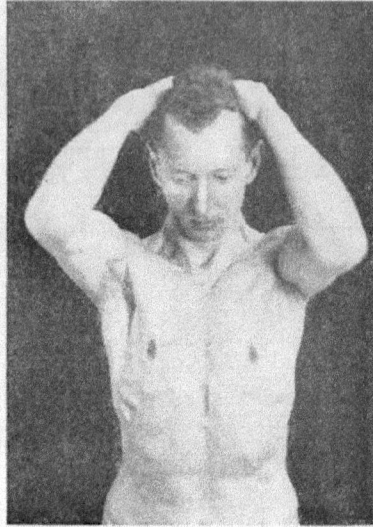

Fig. 1 B.

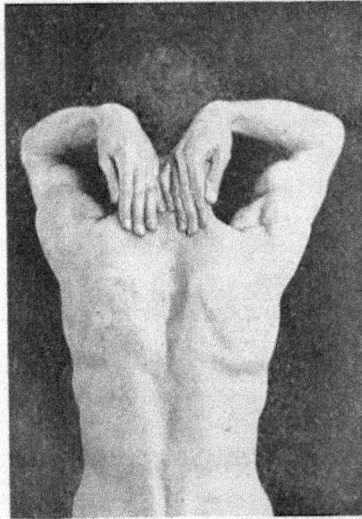

Fig. 1 C.

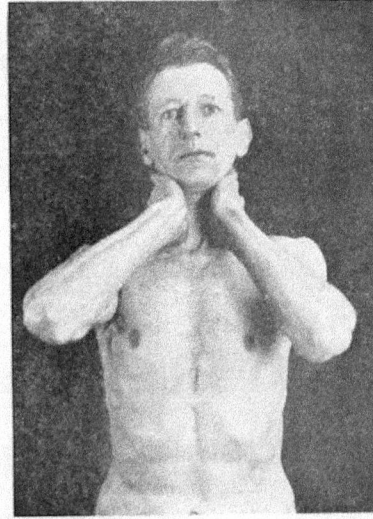

Fig. 1 D.

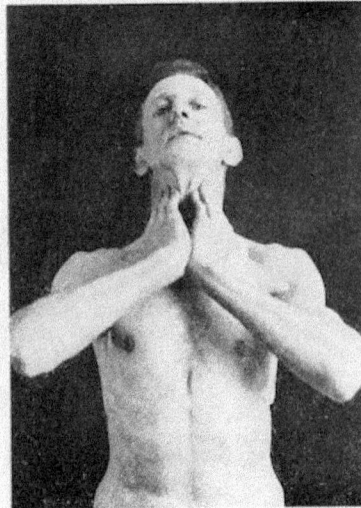

Fig. 1 E.

Fig. 1 A.   Fig. 1 B.

Fig. 1 C.   Fig. 1 D.

Fig. 1 E.

With the four fingers together and the thumbs close, place the inner side of the fingers in the middle of the forehead, so that the hands are nearly parallel to each other (Fig. 1 A). Stroke from there with the fingers and palms of both hands simultaneously up over the head; at the same time bending the head forward (Fig. 1 B). Continue down the back of the head and neck as far as possible, pressing with the fingers on each side of the cervical vertebrae (Fig. 1 C). From here continue the stroking with the palms of the hands and the fingers around each side of the neck toward the throat; at the same time bending the head slowly backward (Fig. 1 D). When the fingers reach the throat they stroke downward on each side of it (Fig. 1 E).

Doing this exercise five times will take about half a minute.

Note I. While the fingers are stroking the neck on each side of the cervical vertebrae, the elbows should be elevated as high as possible.

Note II. Inhale while the hands are moving over the head and down the back of the neck. Exhale while the hands and fingers are moving around the neck and over the throat.

Note III. Women with long and abundant hair, which in hanging loose might interfere with the movements of the hands and fingers, can braid it at the back of the head (pigtail fashion) and the fingers can stroke around each side of it. Or the loosened hair may be parted in the middle, thus leaving the back of the neck comparatively free.

Analysis and Effects of the Combined Massage Exercise No. 1

The influence of the massage movements on the muscles, nerves, tissues and circulation as well as on the internal organs has already been described to some extent in the Chapter, "Construction and Characteristics of the Combined Massage Exercises." Therefore, the analysis and effects of this and the other exercises will only attempt to explain how each exercise is combined, and what nerves, muscles and organs are influenced by it.

This exercise is combined in such a way, that there is obtained the movements of the arms and the bending of the head forward and backward, together with the massage of the temples, the forehead, the scalp, the cervical vertebrae, the neck and the throat.

The movements of the head, arms and hands in applying the massage movements, exercise the muscles and nerves of the hands, arms, shoulders, the upper back, the sides and the chest. They also stretch the muscles and nerves of the latter two.

The massage influences the muscles, vessels, nerves and tissues of the temples, scalp, neck, throat and likewise the glands in the neck.

This exercise acts as a preventive to, and is beneficial for headache, facial neuralgia, falling hair and a disordered circulation to the head. It will reduce fat shoulders and necks and will build up thin ones.

It is also beneficial for singers and public speakers.

THE COMBINED MASSAGE EXERCISE No. 2

Massaging each arm and side alternately from the wrist along the upper aspect of the arm up over shoulder to the base of the neck, then from the wrist again along the under side of the arm over armpit and part of shoulder blade down the same side of body and across the lower chest to the opposite side; at the same time exercising the arms and shoulders.

Detailed Description

Position.—Standing or sitting erect in a bed or chair.

EXERCISE No. 2.

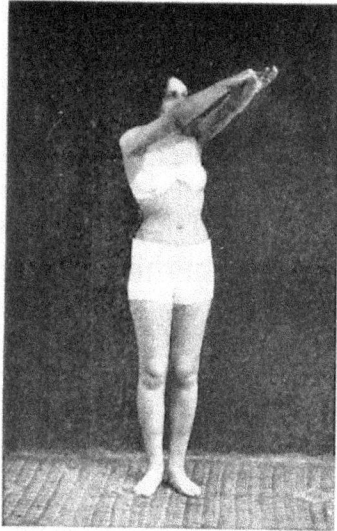

Fig. 2 A.

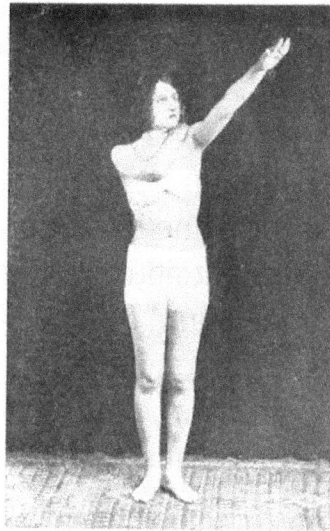

Fig. 2 B.

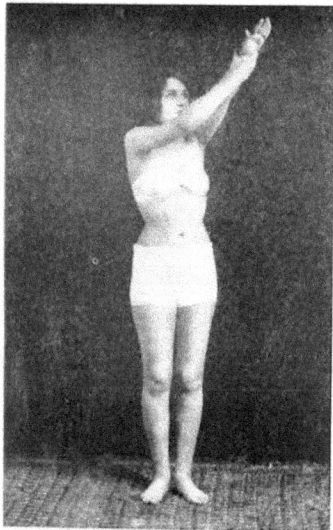

Fig. 2 C.

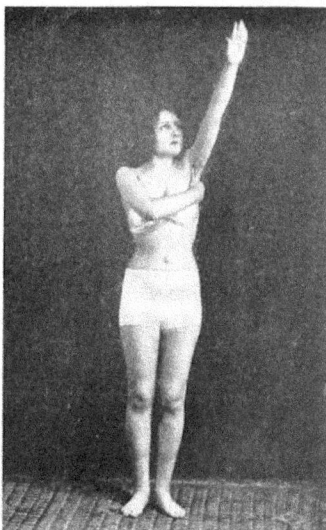

Fig. 2 D.

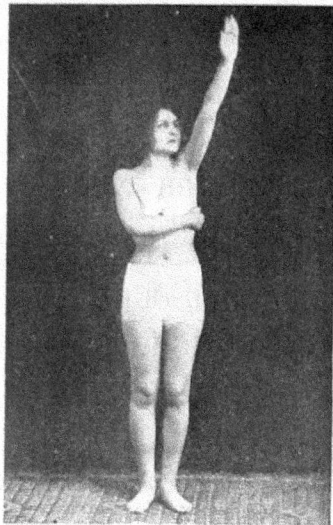

Fig. 2 E.

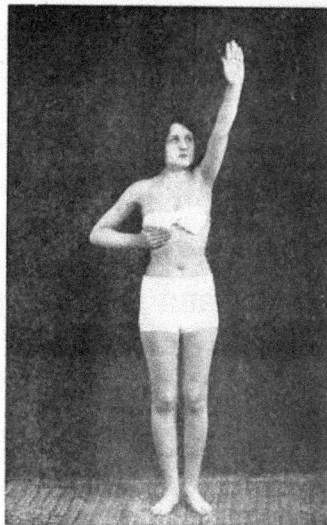

Fig. 2 F.

Fig. 2 A.   Fig. 2 B.

Fig. 2 C.   Fig. 2 D.

Fig. 2 E.   Fig. 2 F.

Stretch the left arm to the front, holding it at such an angle that the tip of the fingers are at the same height or slightly higher than the top of the head, the fingers held straight and together, with the thumbs close. Place the right hand, with the fingers and thumb close, over the upper side of the left arm at or on the wrist in such a way that the hand and fingers are bent transversely over the arm, and so that the palm of the hand and fingers are pressing equally on top and both sides of same (Fig. 2 A).

Stroke thus from there along the upper side of the outstretched arm, continuing over shoulder to the base of the neck (Fig. 2 B). Then let the hand slip loosely backward the same way over the arm to the wrist. Now clutch the out-stretched arm underneath at the wrist in such a way that the thumb is on the inner side and the four fingers on the outer side of the arm (Fig. 2 C). Stroke thus the out-stretched arm underneath from the wrist up to the armpit, at the same time raising it slowly to a nearly perpendicular position. Then continue downward underneath the shoulder with the four fingers around as far as possible on the shoulder blade, and the thumb in the armpit (Fig. 2 D). Continue downward the same side of body, the fingers being kept as far over toward the back as possible and the hand held transversely to the side of the body and bent in such a way that it presses equally with the palm and the fingers. When the hand has thus passed just below a line horizontal to the nipple of the left breast (Fig. 2 E) let it move across the chest underneath the nipples to the other side, in that way, thus not altering the position of the hand itself (Fig. 2 F).

During this massage of the left side and across the lower chest, the left arm should still be held in its out-stretched position over the head.

Upon completing the movement on the right side and changing to the left, release the right hand from the chest and put out the right arm, holding it in the same position as was the left, in the beginning. At the same time let the left arm be brought down with its hand on the upper side of the right wrist and begin to stroke the right arm and side in the same manner as the left. In thus changing from one arm and side to the other, practically no stop should be made.

NOTE I. When the upper side of one of the arms has been massaged to the base of the neck, it is not absolutely necessary to let the hand go back over the arm, as described, in order to massage it underneath. The hand can simply be taken away from the neck and the outstretched arm grasped underneath the wrist without touching its upper side. However, it is best performed in the way first described, but let the hands return, barely touching the arm.

Analysis and Effects of the Combined Massage Exercise No. 2

This exercise is combined in such a way that there is obtained the movements of the arms together with their massage and that of the shoulders, the sides of the upper body, the outer sides of the upper back, and the lower chest.

The arms and shoulders are here exercised to a greater extent than in exercise No. 1. Thus, for instance, if the left arm is being stroked upward with the right hand, the muscles of the right hand are not only exercised, but likewise those of the left arm and shoulder, the latter are especially put into play because the left arm is resisting the pressure of the right hand upon it. The left arm furthermore is massaged at the same time. The reverse is of course the case when the right arm is massaged.

The movements of the arms and hands, in applying the massage movements, exercise the muscles and nerves of the hands, the arms, the shoulders, the upper back, the sides, and the lower chest.

The massage influences the muscles, nerves, blood and lymph vessels of the arms, the shoulders, the sides and the lower chest. It also stimulates the action of the liver and strengthens that of the heart.

This exercise is especially beneficial for stiffness in arms and shoulders caused by playing baseball, golf, hockey or from other over-exertion. It will reduce fat shoulders and arms and build up thin ones.

THE COMBINED MASSAGE EXERCISE No. 3

Massaging each leg alternately with both hands simultaneously from ankle upward over leg and hip, continuing from there with one hand above the other and parallel to each other, directly across the abdomen, one hand moving underneath the ribs, over the transverse colon and the stomach and the other hand over the lower abdomen and pelvis; at the same time lifting and stretching the legs and bending the trunk forward and backward.

Detailed Description

Position.—Standing erect with feet parallel and about four inches apart.

EXERCISE No. 3.

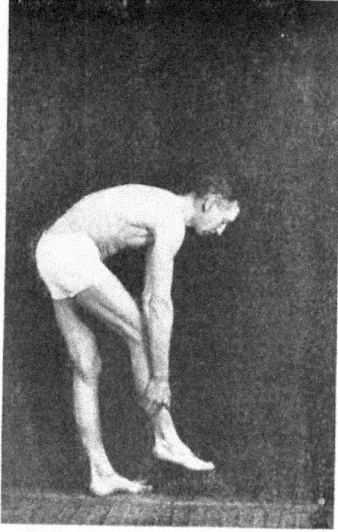

Fig. 3 A.

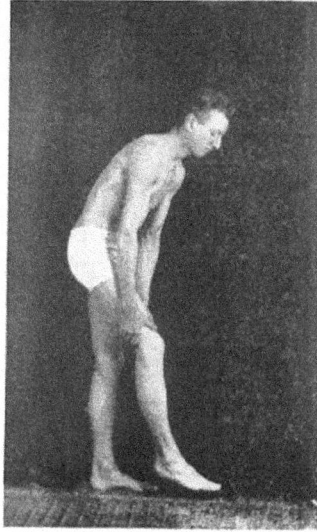

Fig. 3 B.

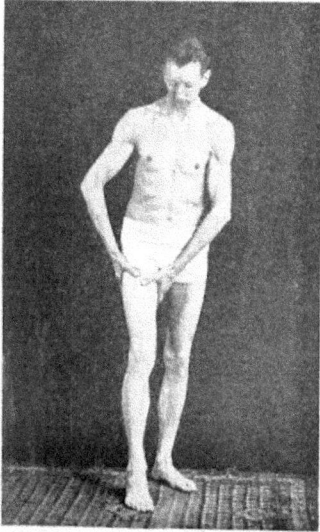

Fig. 3 C.

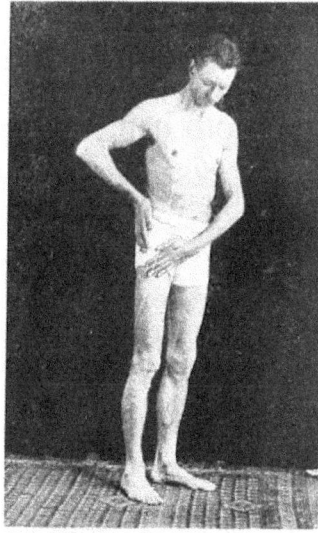

Fig. 3 D.

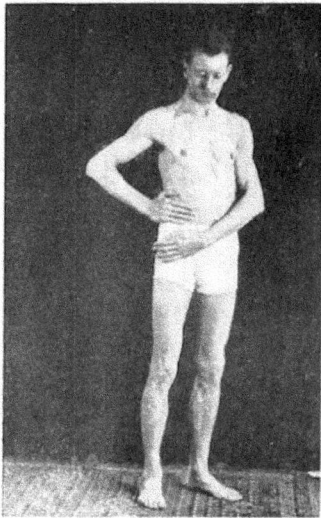

Fig. 3 E.

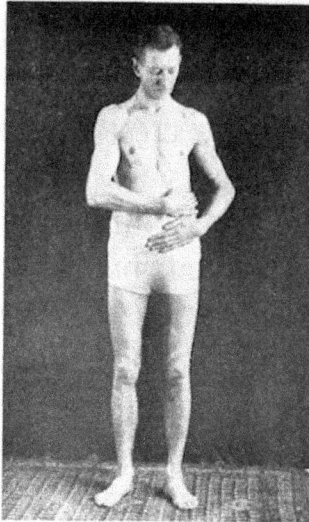

Fig. 3 F.

Fig. 3 A.   Fig. 3 B.

Fig. 3 C.   Fig. 3 D.

Fig. 3 E.   Fig. 3 F.

Bend the trunk forward, at the same time raising the right leg about four inches from the floor, so that it is slightly bent at the knee and hip and pointed somewhat forward. The weight will then rest on the left leg, the knee of which should be held as rigidly as possible. With the trunk bent forward, clutch the right leg with both hands just above the ankle in such a way, that the thumbs are in front on either side of the tibia (shin-bone). The fingers of each hand, which are kept close together are slanted downward and around the back of the leg from each side, so that the third and fourth fingers of each hand meet and touch at the middle line of the calf muscles. The palms of the hands are thus on each side of the leg, the right hand being on the right or outer side and the left on the inner or left side (Fig. 3 A).

Stroke thus with both hands simultaneously from the ankle upward over the lower right leg pressing the muscles with the thumbs and especially with the inner side of the tips of the fingers on the middle of the calf muscles.

While continuing over the knee and in order to conform the hands to the shape of the thigh, turn the thumbs more transversely over the upper side of the thigh and do the same with the fingers underneath, so that as far as possible the muscles of the thigh are influenced all around (Fig. 3 B).

The hands thus reach the groin (Fig. 3 C).

Here the right hand, the fingers pointed downward and thumb close, continues upward over the side of the hip, until the back part of the right palm is just above the crest of the ilium, or hip bone. Here it is turned around so that the fingers are pointing straight toward the left, or toward the middle line of the body. Simultaneously the left hand, at the inner side of the groin, is also turned, but in such a way that the fingers are pointed toward the right and with the back part of the palm it presses and strokes a short distance over the appendix and the lower right side of the abdomen. This is done at the same time as the right hand is stroking upward over the hip and turned around as described (Fig. 3 D). When both hands are thus turned, the left will be underneath the right, the fingers of each hand pointed in an opposite direction and the hands parallel to each other. The right foot is placed on the floor, at the time that the hands reach the groin or hip, and at the same time, the upper body is returned to an upright position, the shoulders thrown slightly backward without strain. The abdominal muscles should be neither distended nor contracted, but kept in a natural position (Fig. 3 E).

Without bending the body to sides, continue thus with both hands simultaneously across the abdomen, the right hand with fingers first, moves underneath the ribs, and pressure is exerted with the fingers and palm over the abdominal viscera (the point of the liver, the transverse colon, the region of the solar plexus, the duodenum, the pylorus, and the stomach) and finishes over on the left side, with the fingers moving between the crest of the ilium, or hip bone, and the lowest border of the ribs. The left hand with the back of the palm preceding, at the same time strokes across the lower abdomen just underneath the umbilicus or navel, and over to the left side, where it is released simultaneously with the right hand (Fig. 3 F).

Now stroke over the left leg, hip and abdomen in a similar way, but of course with this difference; that here the left hand strokes upward over the outer side of the leg, over the left hip and across the stomach from the left, above the right hand. The latter moves from the inner side of the leg, across the lower abdomen below the left hand. In other words, the left hand massages over the left leg and side and from the latter across the abdomen in the same way as the right hand does on the right side, and likewise the right hand massages over the left leg and side and from the latter across the abdomen, in the same way as does the left hand on the right side.

This exercise done five times will take about half a minute. If counting each time when commencing to stroke each leg it will be ten counts.

NOTE I. The raising of the trunk should be the force, which here pulls the arms and hands over the leg.

NOTE II. In bending to massage upward on each leg, the latter can also be bent and raised as high as possible. In that case the leg is pushed downward through the hands, while these are pressing on it, the muscles of the thigh or hip thus being exercised and influenced more than if the leg is raised or bent only a short distance. On the contrary, if the leg is placed only slightly forward with but little flexion of the knee, as explained in the detailed description, the upper body has to be bent further downward in order that the hands reach the lower leg at the ankle. In this way, the muscles of the abdomen and back are exercised and influenced to a greater extent.

If the exercise is done only five times it should be executed as explained in the *Detailed Description*; if done ten times or more, both ways may be used about an equal number of times each.

Exercise No. 3 A

Position.—Lying supine on the floor or bed.

EXERCISE NO. 3A.

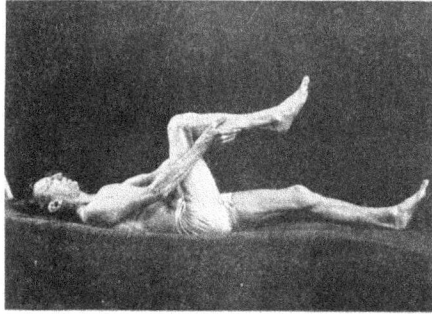

Fig. 3A—A.

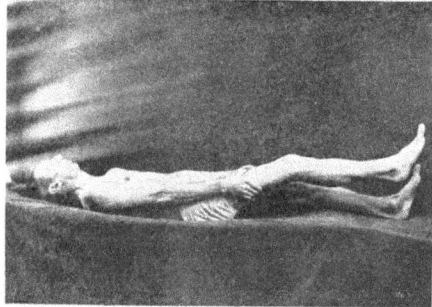

Fig. 3A—B.

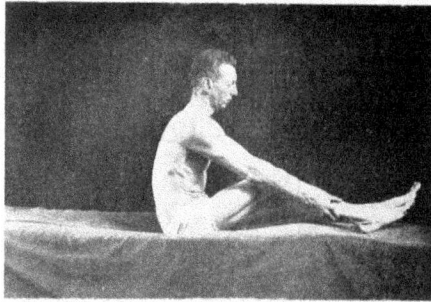

Fig. 3A—C.

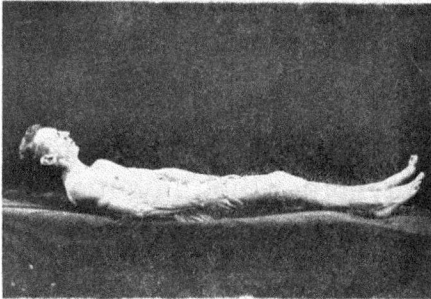

Fig. 3A—D.

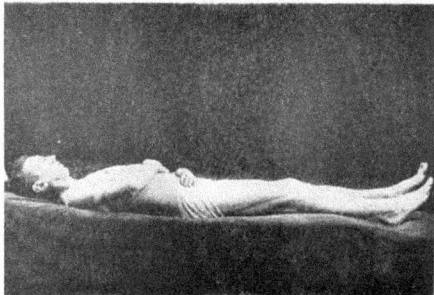

Fig. 3A—E.

Fig. 3A—A.

Fig. 3A—B.

Fig. 3A—C.

Fig. 3A—D.

Fig. 3A—E.

Here the movements are the same as in No. 3, except that they are done from the position of lying flat on the back on a bed or mattress. Those of the leg and trunk may be altered in a similar way to those of No. 3. Thus the upper body can remain resting with the back on the bed, while each leg is bent up and firmly held with the hands at the ankle. The leg then pushes itself through them (Fig. 3 A—A and B).

Or, the upper body can be raised and each leg kept nearly straight or bent more or less, is then stroked while the trunk is being bent backward and downward again on the bed (similar to a rowing exercise) (Fig. 3 A—C and D).

The leg and trunk should be back and resting flat on the bed while the hands are stroking over the hips and abdomen, so that the latter is neither distended nor contracted, but kept in a natural and relaxed position (Fig. 3 A—E).

Analysis and Effects of the Combined Massage Exercise No. 3 (3 A)

This exercise is combined so that there is obtained practically the same movements as in rowing, together with massage of the legs and the abdomen. This is the case whether the movements are done from a standing position or while lying or sitting.

The movements of the legs, the trunk and the arms and hands, in applying the massage movements, exercise the muscles and nerves of the hands, the arms, the shoulders, the back and the sides of the body, the chest, the abdomen and the legs. They also exercise the liver and other digestive organs and have a beneficial influence on the heart. They stretch the nerves in the spine in a natural way.

The massage influences the muscles, nerves and vessels of the legs and the abdomen, also the lower point of the liver, the pancreas, the stomach, the intestines, the different abdominal nerve-plexuses, the appendix and the organs of the pelvis. The heart is influenced indirectly through the circulation of the blood.

This exercise is beneficial for pain and weakness in the legs, caused by diseased conditions of the nerves, as in sciatica, partial paralysis, etc. (See Supplement, page 92.) It is especially beneficial for disorders in the digestive system, as in chronic or habitual constipation, gas in the stomach, etc. (See Supplement, page 88). It is beneficial to the generative organs in women. It is especial beneficial for professional dancers and runners and people whose profession causes great strain on the legs.

It should be remembered that in this and all the other exercises where the abdominal organs are massaged, it is important not to let the hands go over the ribs and the upper abdominal cavity at the same time. The digestive organs cannot be properly reached and influenced in this way. Especially is this the case if the hand strokes in a perpendicular position, that is, with fingers pointing downward and not transversely. Even if the hands were stroking over the abdomen, underneath the ribs in a perpendicular position, this would not be sufficient for the reason that as much pressure can not be exerted in this way as with the hands in a transverse position. It would also cover too many organs at one time to make a sufficient impression upon them.

THE COMBINED MASSAGE EXERCISE No. 4

Massaging each side alternately from the side of the knee upward over the thigh, hip and side, then across the lower chest or underneath the breasts, to the opposite side; and at the same time bending the upper body from side to side.

Detailed Description

Position.—Standing erect with shoulders thrown backward and chest forward, but without strain, heels together and feet and legs stationary.

EXERCISE No. 4.

EXERCISE NO. 4.

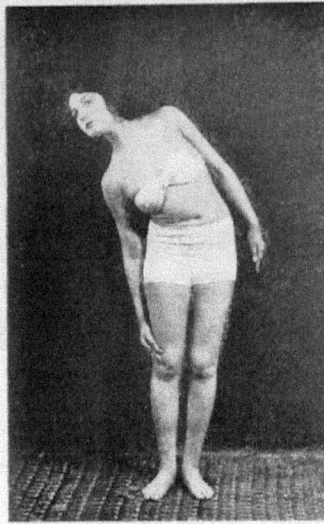

Fig. 4 A.

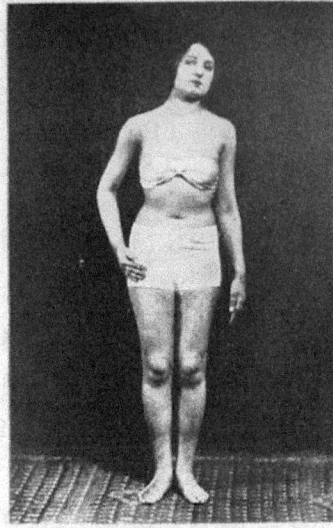

Fig. 4 B.

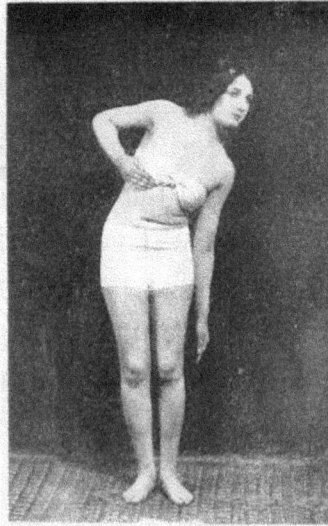

Fig. 4 C.

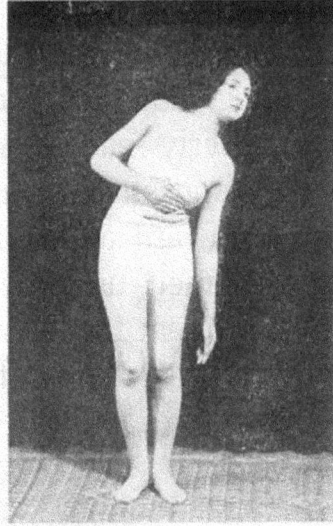

Fig. 4 D.

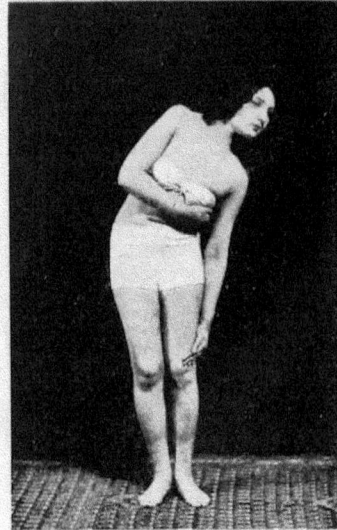

Fig. 4 E.

Fig. 4 A.   Fig. 4 B.

Fig. 4 C.   Fig. 4 D.

Fig. 4 E.

Without altering the position of the legs, bend the upper body to the right as far as possible, so that the right hand is level with or just above the outer side of the right knee. Place this hand, with fingers and thumb close, transversely over the side of the thigh just above the knee so that the fingers are pointing inward, toward the left (Fig. 4 A).

Stroke thus with the right hand from there upward over the side of the right thigh, hip and trunk until the thumb is horizontal with the nipple of the right breast, the fingers of the hand should thus be pointing straight toward the left side. In thus stroking upward on the right side the trunk should be bent directly to the left (Fig. 4 B and C).

Then without altering the position of the body or the hand, continue stroking with the latter, fingers first, across the lower chest over the region of the liver under the right nipple of the breast, toward the left side (Fig. 4 D), where the hand moves underneath the nipple of the breast, over the lower region of the heart and is released on that side (Fig. 4 E).

Now alternate to the left side. The upper body is still bent to the left, and the left hand is placed on the side of the left thigh, just above the knee (Fig. 4 E). Now massage the left thigh, hip and side and from there across the chest with the left hand, in the same way as the right side was massaged with the right hand. When the hand is moving upward over the left thigh, hip and side, the body is of course bent to the right. After the left side has been massaged, repeat the movements on the right and so forth, alternately.

This exercise done five times will take about fifteen seconds. If counting every time when commencing to stroke from each side of hip, it will be ten counts.

Analysis and Effects of the Combined Massage Exercise No. 4

This exercise is combined in such a manner that there is obtained the movements of the arms and the bending of the body sideways, together with massage of the outer side of the thighs, the hips, the sides of the body and the lower chest.

The movements of the body and arms and hands in applying the massage movements, exercise the muscles and nerves of the arms, the shoulders, the back, the sides, the lower chest and breasts and the abdomen. They also slightly influence the liver, the stomach, the intestines and kidneys.

The massage influences the muscles, nerves and vessels of the outer side of the thighs, the hips, the lower sides of the trunk and the lower chest, as well as the liver and the heart.

THE COMBINED MASSAGE EXERCISE No. 5

Massaging the right leg with the right hand and the left leg with the left hand simultaneously from behind the ankles upward over the backs and sides of the lower legs, backs and sides of the thighs, continuing a short distance upward over the hips and from there, still with both hands at the same time, across the abdomen and lower chest to the opposite sides, the right hand passing from the right side underneath the ribs over to the left side, and the left hand passing from the left side underneath the nipples or breasts over to the right side. From there, continue stroking with both hands simultaneously inward and upward over the opposite nipples or breasts and the upper chest where the hands pass each other and stroke outward to their respective sides under the armpits; the right hand thus stroking from the left side inward and upward over the left nipple or breast and the left hand from the right side inward and upward over the right nipple or breast. Release the hands at the armpits and stroke down each side of the lower back and buttocks with the backs of the hands. At the same time, bending the upper body forward and backward.

Detailed Description

Position.—Standing erect with heels about eight inches apart and feet nearly parallel.

EXERCISE NO. 5.

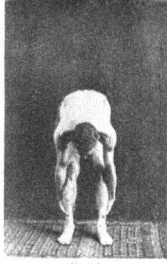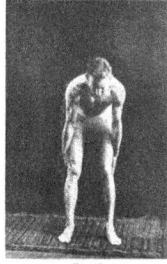

Fig. 3 A.   Fig. 3 B.

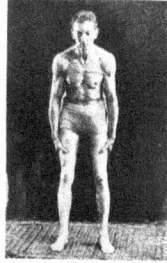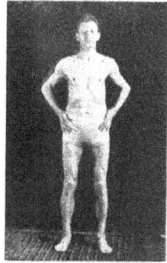

Fig. 3 C.   Fig. 3 D.

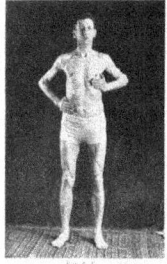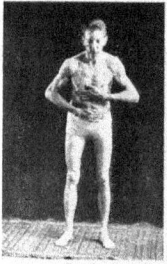

Fig. 3 E.   Fig. 3 F.

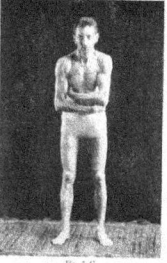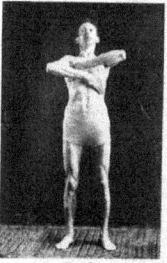

Fig. 3 G.   Fig. 3 H.

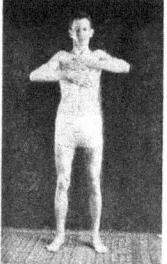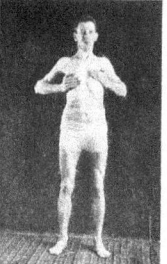

Fig. 3 I.   Fig. 3 J.

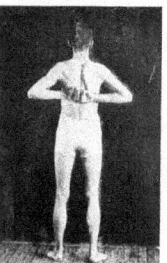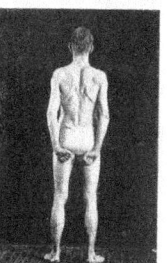

Fig. 3 K.   Fig. 3 L.

Fig. 5 A.	Fig. 5 B.
Fig. 5 C.	Fig. 5 D.
Fig. 5 E.	Fig. 5 F.
Fig. 5 G.	Fig. 5 H.
Fig. 5 I.	Fig. 5 J.
Fig. 5 K.	Fig. 5 L.

Without bending the legs, bend the upper body forward as far as possible, and clutch the lower right leg with the right hand and the lower left leg with the left hand from behind and just above the ankles in such a way that the palm of each hand is on the back of each leg, the four fingers placed around the inner sides and thumbs around the outer sides, thus making an equal pressure with fingers and palms of hands around each leg (Fig. 5 A).

Now, stroke upward over the calf muscles and thighs, the palms of the hands here stroking the outer sides of the latter, the four fingers underneath and the thumb on top, at the same time raising the trunk to an upright position (Fig. 5 B and C).

While the hands continue upward over the sides of hips, turn them around so that the fingers point inward (Fig. 5 D). Continue thus with the right hand on the right side until it is just above the crest of the ilium, or hip bone. The left hand, at the same time moves a little higher upward on the left side until its thumb is nearly horizontal with the nipple of the left breast. The trunk is now in an upright position, the shoulders thrown well back (Fig. 5 E).

With the fingers of both hands thus pointing toward the middle of the body, continue stroking with both hands simultaneously from each side across the front of the body, to the opposite sides, the left hand above the right, passing each other at the middle line. Bend the trunk slightly forward at the same time (Fig. 5 F). In other words, the right hand strokes from the right side underneath the ribs directly over to the left side, above the crest of the left ilium, or hip bone, and around as far as possible on that side. The left hand strokes at the same time from the left side across the lower chest, underneath the nipples over to and around as far as possible on the right side. The left forearm is thus crossed over the right (Fig. 5 G).

Then continue stroking with both hands simultaneously from each side inward and upward over each breast and upper chest. The right hand thus moving from the left side strokes inward and upward over the left breast and across the upper chest to the right side and ceases underneath the right armpit. The left hand moving from the right side, strokes inward and upward over the right breast and across the upper chest to the left side and ceases under the left armpit. At the same time, the trunk which has been bent slightly forward, while the hands were stroking across the lower chest and abdomen, is raised and bent slightly backward. In thus stroking inward and upward over the chest, the hands and fingers are held in the same way as when they were on the sides of the body. When moving over the breasts the left forearm is of course crossed over the right (Fig. 5 H), but when reaching the middle of the chest the hands cross, the left hand being directly above the right (Fig. 5 I), and from there they continue stroking transversely over the chest to their respective sides under the armpit (Fig. 5 J).

The hands are now released and brought as far up on the back as possible. The backs of the clenched hands are placed on each side of the back, in such a way, that the knuckles at the base of the finger of each hand are close to and opposite each other on each side of the spinal column (Fig. 5 K). Stroke thus from there with the backs of both hands simultaneously downward on each side of the lower back and buttocks, the knuckles following the spine on each side of same (Fig. 5 L).

This exercise done five times will take about half a minute.

Note I. If unable to place the hands behind the ankles without bending the knees, the latter may be bent slightly or the leg stroked at a distance from the ankle possible to reach without bending the knees.

Note II. When the hands are stroking and pressing over the legs, let the raising movement of the trunk pull the out-stretched arms up as far as the motion permits.

Combined with Deep Breathing

If done very slowly, deep breathing may be practiced with this exercise in the following way: Inhale the air through the nose, while stroking upward over the legs and hips and raising the upper body.

Exhale this air through the mouth while stroking and pressing across the body from sides, and while the upper body is being bent slightly forward.

Inhale again through the nose, while stroking inward and upward over the chest, and while the upper body is being again bent upward and slightly backward.

Retain this air in the lungs while the hands are moving down the spine, back and buttocks.

Exhale this air through the mouth, while the body is being bent downward, in order to repeat the exercise.

If special or general deep breathing exercises are practiced between each massage exercise, natural breathing during this exercise will be sufficient. In the event that the reader has little available time and may wish to practice some deep breathing and exercises for a few minutes, this combination will be found admirable.

Analysis and Effects of the Combined Massage Exercise No. 5

This exercise is so combined that there is obtained the movements of the arms and the bending of the trunk forward and backward together with massage of the back and sides of the legs, the hips, the sides of the upper body, the chest and breasts, the abdomen and lower back, and the buttocks.

The movements of the trunk, arms and hands, in applying the massage movements, exercise the muscles and nerves of the arms, the shoulders and the entire upper body, including the abdomen. The organs of the latter are influenced in the same way. The muscles of the legs are here not exercised to the same extent as in exercise No. 3, but if the legs are kept straight in bending the trunk forward the great sciatic and other nerves of the leg are stretched in a natural way. The spinal cord is also stretched.

The massage influences the legs, but not to such an extent as in exercise No. 3, first, because each is here only massaged with one hand and secondly, because the muscles are kept more rigid by the bending of the body, for the reason that the weight of the body is upon them. It influences the muscles, nerves and vessels of the abdomen, the hips, the sides, the chest and breasts, the lower and upper back and especially the spine and the buttocks. It also influences the heart, the liver both from in front and behind, and the kidneys. It influences the digestive organs directly from in front and indirectly through the nerves in the back.

To call attention to the difference between scientific massage movements and rubbing, it may be pointed out that there are five principal massage movements combined with the movements of the body in this exercise, namely:

1. The stroking and pressing upward over the back of the legs.

2. The manner in which the right hand strokes and presses directly across the abdomen from the right.

3. The stroking and pressing with the left hand from the left side over the region of the heart to the opposite side.

4. The stroking and pressing with the hands from each opposite side of the lower chest, over the region of the heart and liver inward and upward across the chest.

5. The manner in which the backs of the clutched hands are stroking and pressing downward on each side of the lower back and the spine.

If the hands would stroke over the front of the lower legs and continue straight up over the abdomen and then downward on the backs of the legs instead of upwards; neither the nerves, muscles and vessels of the legs nor the internal organs would be influenced in the proper way. Such rubbing would be of little value.

THE COMBINED MASSAGE EXERCISE No. 6

Massaging with both hands simultaneously downward on each side of back and buttocks; at the same time turning the trunk to the right and left.

Detailed Description

Position.—Standing erect with chest thrown forward and shoulders back, but without strain, heels about five inches apart and with the feet either pointed slightly outward to each side or parallel to each other, arms hanging loosely at side.

EXERCISE NO. 6.

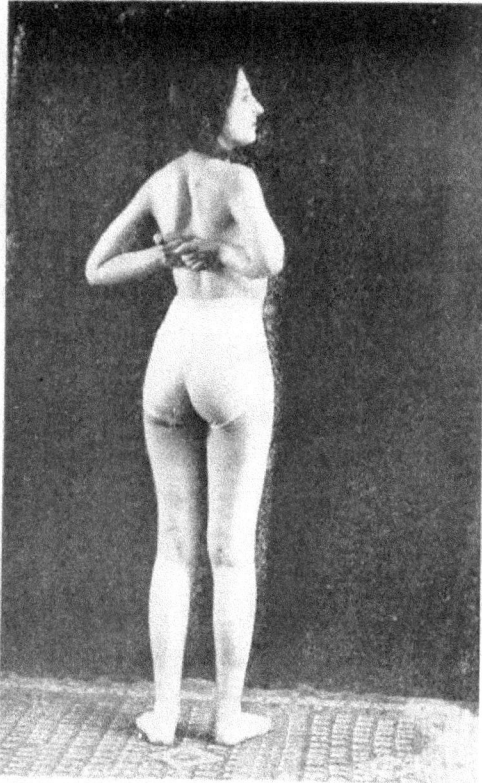

Fig. 6 A.

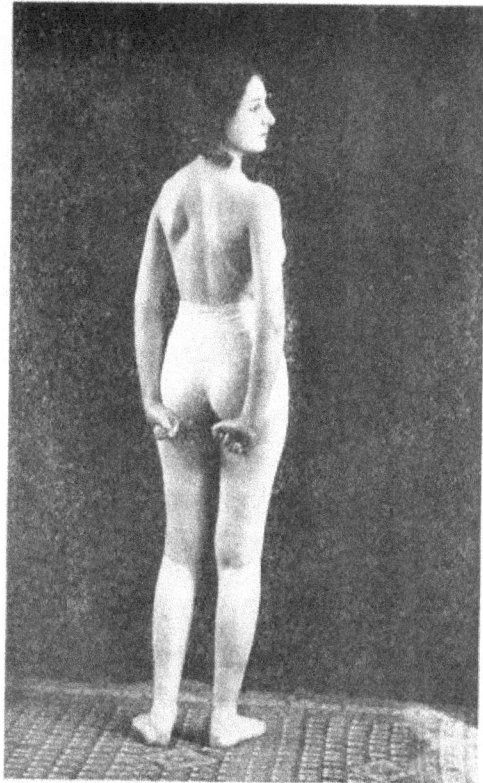

Fig. 6 B.

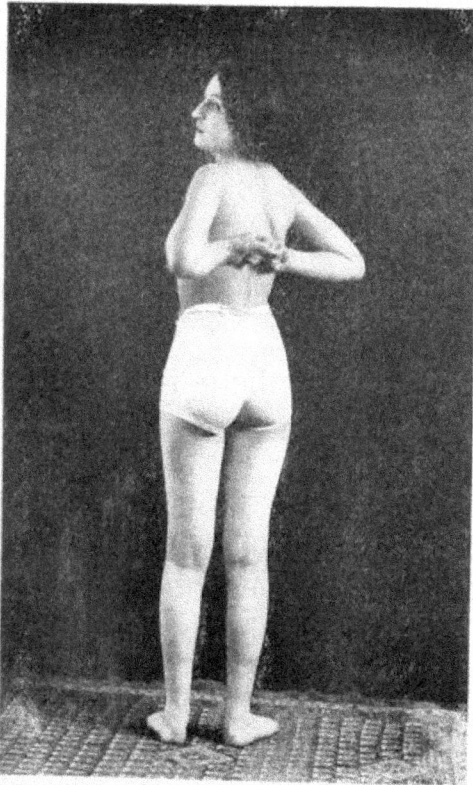

Fig. 6 C.

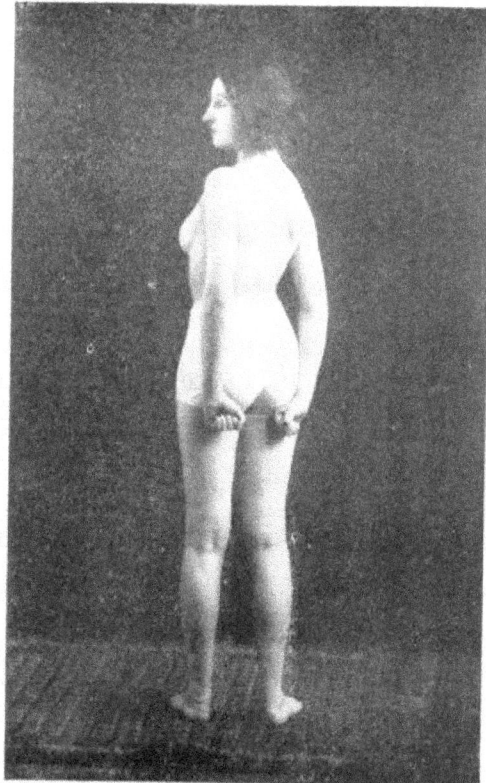

Fig. 6 D.

Fig. 6 A.   Fig. 6 B.

Fig. 6 C.   Fig. 6 D.

Without altering the position of legs and feet, turn the trunk around to the right so that if possible the chest and shoulders are facing squarely to that side. The trunk will thus have made a quarter of a turn to the right. While the body is in that position, clench the hands and move them quickly around and as far up as possible on each side of the back, the back of the hands turned toward the body, the knuckles of each hand opposite each other on each side of the spinal column (Fig. 6 A).

Stroke thus with the backs of both hands simultaneously downward over each side of the lower back and buttocks, where the hands are released (Fig. 6 B).

Now, without altering the position of the legs or feet, turn the trunk over to the left side, as far as possible, so that the chest and shoulders are facing squarely to the left. Thus this time a half turn is made. While in this position, stroke downward on the back in the same way as when the body was turned toward the other side (Fig. 6 C and D).

Alternate by turning to the right, that is, half a turn from the last posture, etc.

This exercise done five times will take about ten seconds. If counting every time the trunk is turned to the side, it will be ten counts.

Analysis and Effects of the Combined Massage Exercise No. 6

This exercise is combined in such a way that there is obtained the movements of the arms and the turning of the upper body to each side, together with massage of the lower back and buttocks.

The movements of the body and the arms and hands in applying the massage movements exercise the muscles and nerves of the arms, the shoulders, the upper chest, the upper and lower back, the hips and the sides of the body. They also influence the kidneys.

The massage influences the muscles, nerves and vessels of the lower back and buttocks, and also the kidneys, bladder and liver and, through the back, the nerves leading to the abdominal organs.

THE COMBINED MASSAGE EXERCISE No. 7

With the exception of the vibratory-pushing-movements of the tissues over the region of the heart and liver and a new arm movement, this exercise is a combination of some of the most important movements of other exercises in this volume, which are here executed in a different order. This is done, first, to get one of the most important and concentrated exercises in the middle of the course, and secondly, so that it can be used when there is time for only one or two exercises, thus serving the benefit of as many of the most important movements as possible, in the shortest time.

Detailed Description

Position.—Standing erect.

EXERCISE NO. 7.

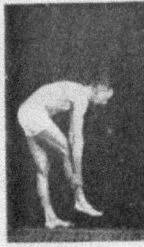 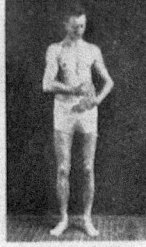 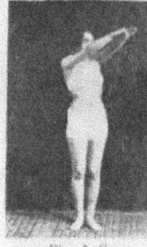 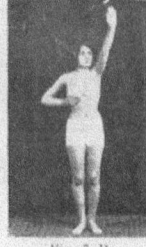

Fig. 7 A.   Fig. 7 B.   Fig. 7 C.   Fig. 7 D.

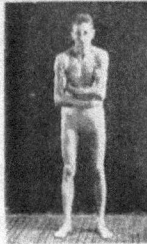 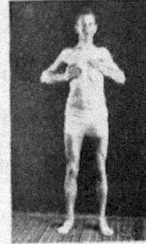 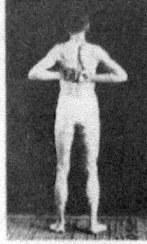 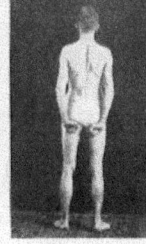

Fig. 7 E.   Fig. 7 F.   Fig. 7 G.   Fig. 7 H.

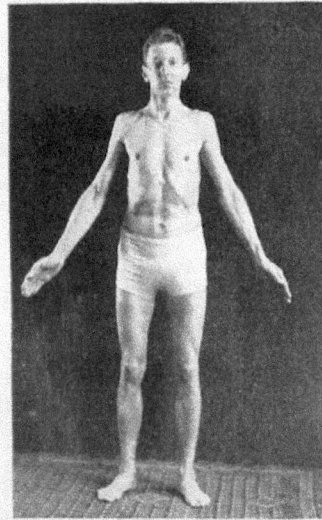 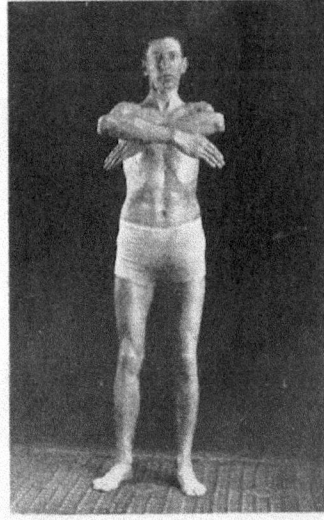

Fig. 7 I.   Fig. 7 J.

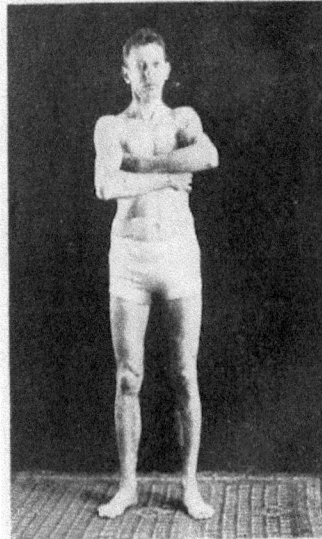 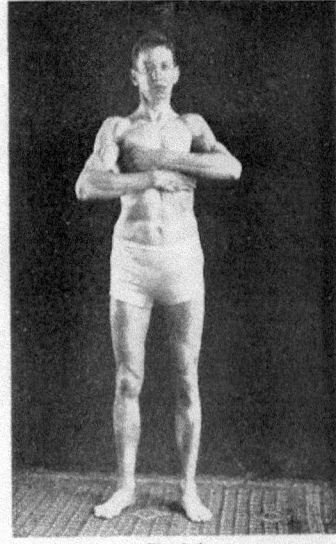

Fig. 7 K.   Fig. 7 L.

Fig. 7 A.   Fig. 7 B.   Fig. 7 C.   Fig. 7 D.

Fig. 7 E.   Fig. 7 F.   Fig. 7 G.   Fig. 7 H.

Fig. 7 I.   Fig. 7 J.

Fig. 7 K.   Fig. 7 L.

Massage upward over the right leg and side of hip and from there across the abdomen to the left side, as in exercise No. 3 (Fig. 7 A and B) or (Fig. 3 A to F).

Release the hands there and massage the right arm and side and across the lower chest with the left hand as in exercise No. 2. (*This movement has not been illustrated as it is similar to the massaging of the left arm, side and from there across the lower chest.*)

Release the left hand and massage the left leg and across the abdomen as in exercise No. 3. (*The massaging of the left leg and across the abdomen has likewise not been illustrated as it is similar to the massaging of the right leg and across the abdomen.*)

Release the hands and massage the left arm, left side and over the lower chest as in exercise No. 2 (Fig. 7 C and D) or (Fig. 2 A to F).

Now, bend the upper body, this time only slightly forward and cross the left forearm over the right, thus placing the hands on the opposite lower sides of the trunk and massage from there inward and upward over the breast and upper chest as in exercise No. 5 (Fig. 7 E and F) or (Fig. 5 G to J).

From there let the hands be brought around and stroke down each side of the back and buttocks with the backs of the hands, as in exercise No. 5 (Fig. 7 G and H) or (Fig. 5 K and L).

Now, swing the out-stretched arms around to the front (Fig. 7 I), bend the elbows (Fig. 7 J) and place the palms of the hands, with fingers out-stretched and close together, on each opposite side of the lower chest (Fig. 7 K) and while keeping the hands stationary on the skin, quickly move or push this and the underlying tissues and muscles sideways four times (Fig. 7 L).

This exercise done five times will take about one minute.

Notice—The exercise should, like all the others, be executed so that there is no pause between the various movements.

Combined with Deep Breathing

If the exercise is done slowly, deep breathing may be added in the following way:

Inhale deeply and forcibly through the nose so that the lungs are filled with air, while the hands are moving upward over the right leg and side of hip and the body is being raised.

Exhale this air quickly and forcibly through the mouth, while continuing massage over the abdomen to the left side, with the body bent slightly forward.

Breathe through the nose in the same way, while the left hand strokes the right arm and continues underneath the shoulder.

Exhale this air with force through the mouth, while the hand continues down the right side and from there across the lower chest.

Inhale and exhale when massaging up over the left leg and hip and across the abdomen in the same way as when the right leg and side were massaged.

Inhale and exhale again the same way, while the right arm is massaging the left arm, side and across the lower chest as when the right arm was massaged.

Breathe again with force through the nose, while massaging inward and upward over the chest.

Retain this air in the lungs, while the backs of the hands are stroking downward on each side of the back and buttocks and while the arms are swinging around to the front.

Exhale this air through the mouth, while the hands are vibrating or pushing the skin over the underlying tissues on each opposite side of the lower chest, or on or underneath the breasts. Continue this movement with the hands and do not release them until the lungs are completely emptied of air.

This exercise is combined in such a way that there is obtained the movements of the arms, the bending and stretching of the legs and the bending and raising of the body together with the massage of the arms, sides, legs, hips, abdomen, chest and back.

The movements of the legs, the upper body, the arms and hands in applying the massage movements, exercise the muscles and nerves of the whole body, except those of the head and neck. They influence all the internal organs of the body.

The massage likewise influences the muscles, nerves, glands, vessels and organs of the whole body except those of the head, neck, the middle of the uppermost part of the back and the feet.

The deep breathing profoundly influences the lungs, the blood, the nervous system, the digestive system, the heart, the liver and the respiratory muscles.

THE COMBINED MASSAGE EXERCISE No. 8

Massaging down both sides of the lower back alternately, with the back of each hand; at the same time turning the trunk to the right and left.

Detailed Description

Position.—Standing erect, with chest thrown forward and shoulders back, but without strain, heels about five inches apart and with the feet either pointed slightly outward to each side or parallel to each other, arms hanging loosely at sides.

EXERCISE No. 8.

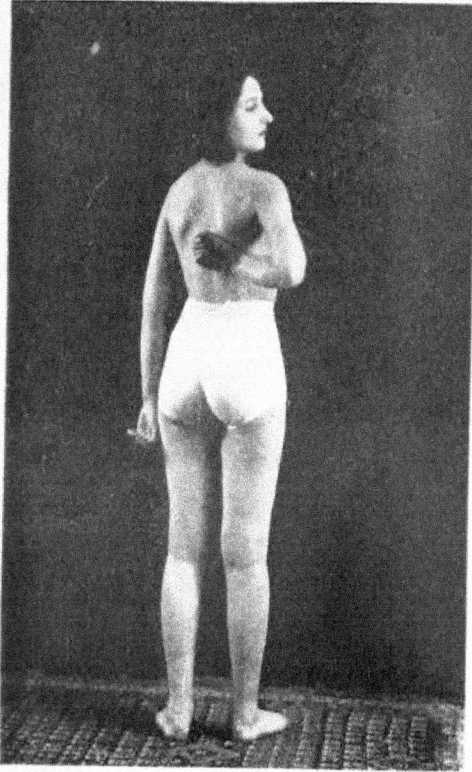

Fig. 8 A.

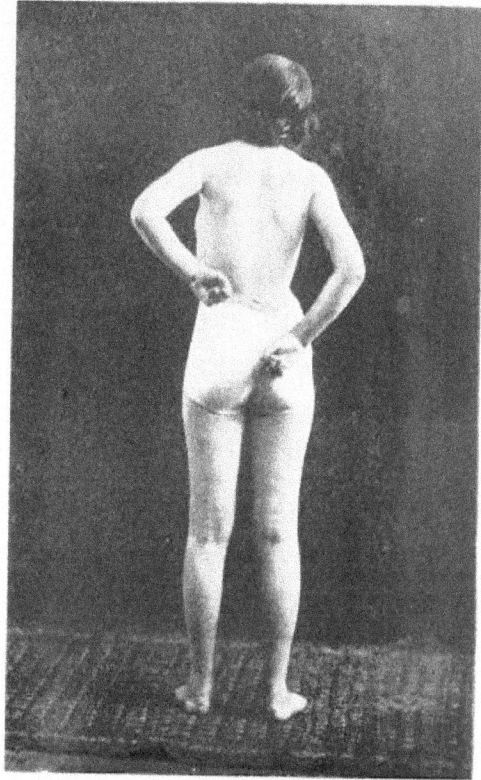

Fig. 8 B.

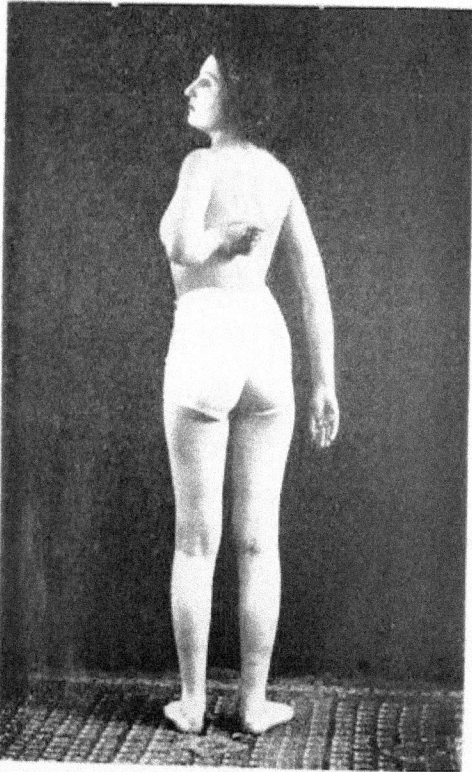

Fig. 8 C.

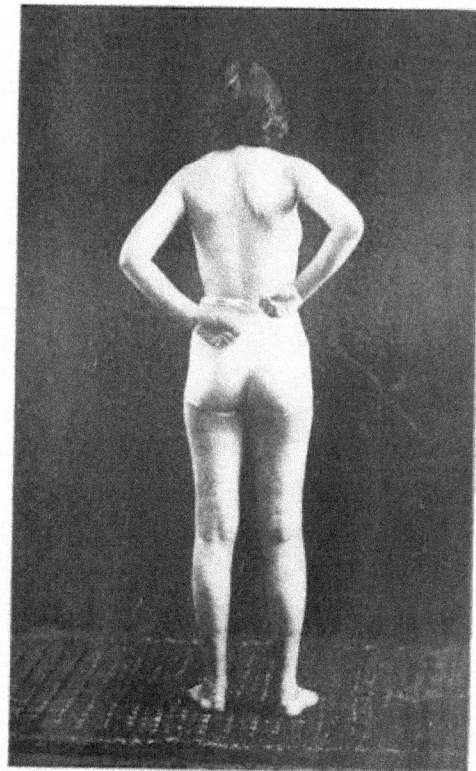

Fig. 8 D.

Fig. 8 A.   Fig. 8 B.

Fig. 8 C.   Fig. 8 D.

Without altering position of legs and feet, turn the trunk around to the right so that, if possible, the chest and shoulders are facing squarely to that side, then turn it to the left, then to the right again, and so forth, alternately. During this movement of the trunk, stroke continually downward over each side of the back from the end of the shoulder blade to the buttocks with the back of each hand alternately. The hands are not clenched, but only half closed. After one stroke is executed that hand is lifted slightly outward from the body and placed underneath the shoulder blade to begin stroking again. The same movement obtains with the opposite hand alternately. Thus the hands come into contact with the tissues only when moving downward on the back (Fig. 8 A, B, C and D). The speed should be about one stroke a second.

This exercise done five times will take about twenty seconds. If counting each time the trunk is turned to either side, it will be ten counts.

Analysis and Effects of the Combined Massage Exercise No. 8

This exercise is combined in such a manner that there is obtained the movements of the arms and the turning of the trunk to each side together with massage of the lower back.

The movements of the body and the arms and hands in applying the massage movements exercise the muscles and nerves of the arms, the shoulders, the upper chest, the upper and lower back, the hips and the sides of the body. They also influence the kidneys.

The massage influences the muscles, nerves and vessels of the lower back. It also influences the kidneys, bladder and liver and, through the back, the nerves leading to the abdominal organs.

THE COMBINED MASSAGE EXERCISE No. 9

Massaging with the right hand from the outer side of the left thigh, upward over the left hip and lower side of trunk, continuing from there, inward and upward over the left nipple or breast and upper chest and across the latter outward to the right armpit. Then, stroking with the left hand from the outer side of the right thigh upward over the right hip and lower side of trunk, and continuing from there, inward and upward over the right nipple or breast and upper chest and across the latter out to the left armpit; at the same time bending the upper body slightly forward and to the right and left.

Detailed Description

Position.—Standing erect, with heels about eight inches apart and feet nearly parallel, legs and feet kept stationary.

Exercise No. 9.

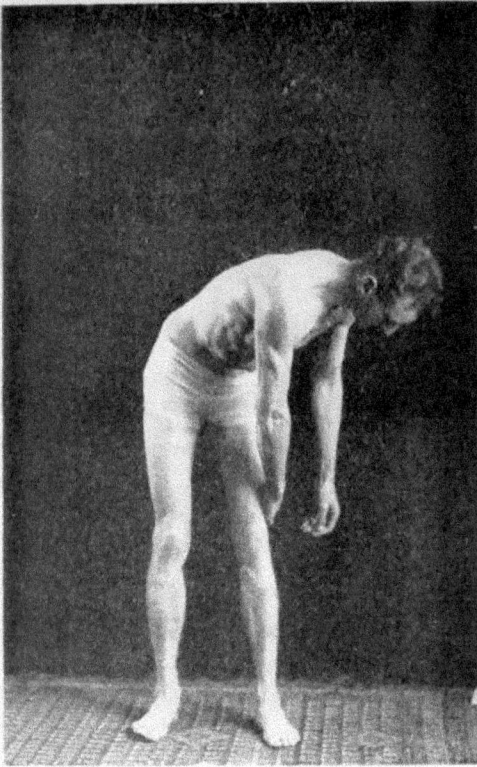

Fig. 9 A.

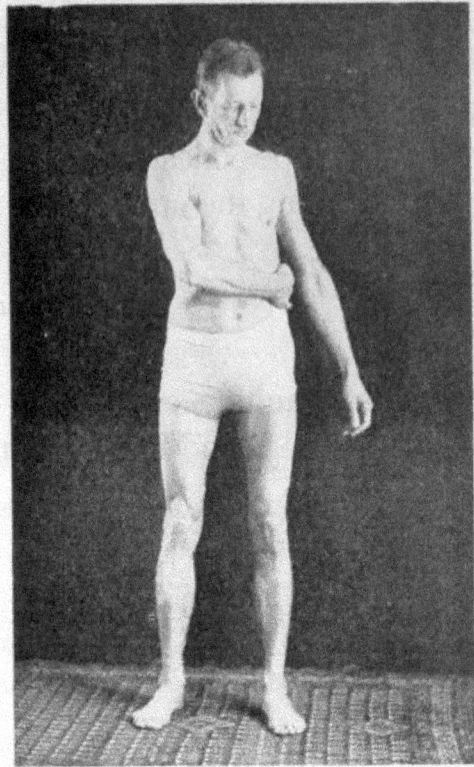

Fig. 9 B.

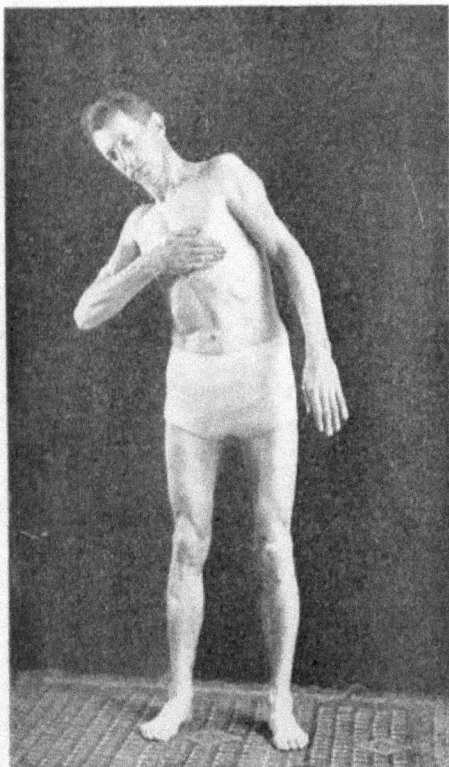

Fig. 9 C.

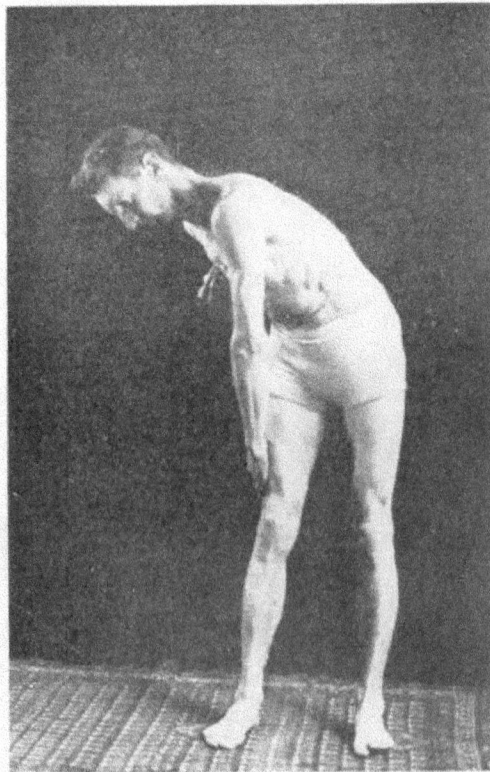

Fig. 9 D.

Fig. 9 A.   Fig. 9 B.

Fig. 9 C.   Fig. 9 D.

Bend the trunk forward and slightly to the left and place the right hand transversely on the outside of the left thigh in such a way that the four fingers are close together and pointed outward and backward (Fig. 9 A).

From there, stroke with the right hand, upward over the side of the left thigh, hip and lower side (Fig. 9 B) and inward and upward over the left nipple or breast and upper chest and outward to the right armpit; at the same time raising the trunk.

When the hand strokes across the upper chest the upper body is bent to the right, but not forward (Fig. 9 C).

Release the right hand at the right armpit; while the upper body is still bent to the right, bend it forward and place the left hand on the outer side of the right thigh (Fig. 9 D) stroking from there upward over the right hip, lower side and inward and upward over the right nipple or breast and upper chest, outward to the left armpit; at the same time raising the upper body. This time, however, the trunk is bent to the left, as the hand strokes the upper chest outward to the left armpit.

Begin again with the right hand on the side of the left thigh and continue thus each side alternately.

This exercise done five times will take about twenty-five seconds. If counting each time when commencing to stroke from the side of the hip, it will be ten counts.

NOTE I. When stroking and pressing upward over the side of each thigh, let the raising movement of the trunk pull the arm and hand up as far as the motion permits.

Exercise No. 9 A

Position.—The same as in exercise No. 9.

Here the same movements are done as in Exercise No. 9, but the following arm exercise has been added:

While the right hand strokes upward over the left side and upper chest, and the body is raised and bent to the right, the left outstretched arm is carried or swung around to the back and upward over the head to the front and down on the outer side of the right thigh, so that it reaches there when the right arm is released at the right armpit. The right arm then performs a similar movement, while the left hand is stroking upward over the right side.

This is somewhat similar to a swimming arm movement. It is also very like the motion used in throwing hand grenades.

NOTE I. Women with well-developed breasts, who might find it somewhat difficult to stroke inward and upward over them, may stroke more or less sideways inward over the breasts, or raise the palm or the back of the hand slightly outward from the body.

Analysis and Effects of the Combined Massage Exercise No. 9 (9 A)

This exercise is combined in such a way that there is obtained the movements of the arms and the bending of the upper body forward and to the sides, together with massage of the outer side of the thighs, the hips, the lower sides of the body, the chest and breasts.

In bending the body forward and to the side, in order to stroke upward over the opposite side from the thigh, the body makes a sort of twisting movement which is especially beneficial for the muscles of the lower sides, the upper abdomen and the lower back, as well as for the liver. These muscles then become stretched when the hand strokes outward to the armpit, on the other side of the upper chest, and the body is bent to that side.

The movements of the body and arms in applying the massage movements, exercise the muscles and nerves of the arms, the shoulders, the back, the chest, the lower sides and the diaphragm. They also influence the liver, the heart and the digestive organs.

The massage influences the muscles of the outer side of the thighs, the hips, the sides of the body and the chest and breasts.

THE COMBINED MASSAGE EXERCISE No. 10

Massaging with the left hand, from the side of the right hip, straight across the lower abdomen to the left side. Then, with the right hand, from the side of the left hip, straight across the lower abdomen to the right side. Massaging again with the left hand from the side of the right hip—but this time with the hand placed about four inches higher up—inward and upward underneath the border of the false ribs to the sternum (the bone in the middle of the chest, and to which the ribs are attached in front). Then massage with the right hand from the side of the left hip inward and upward under the false ribs to the end of the sternum, placing the right hand on top of the left, when massaging with the latter and vice-versa.

Detailed Description

Position.—Standing erect, heels about six inches apart and feet pointed slightly outward, legs and feet stationary.

Exercise No. 10.

EXERCISE No. 10.

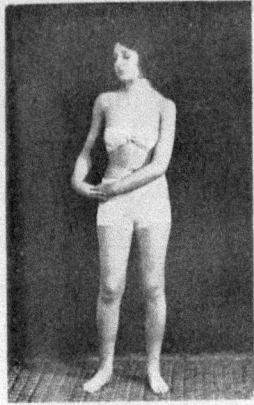

Fig. 10 A.

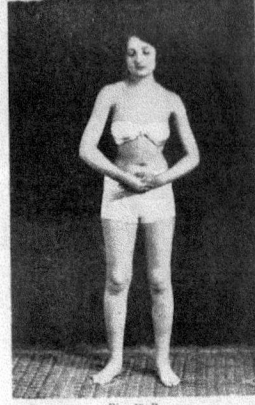

Fig. 10 B.

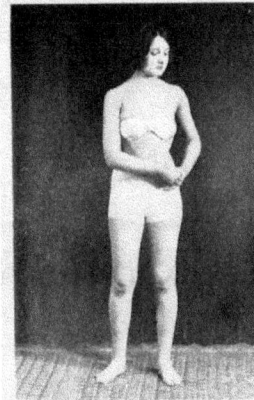

Fig. 10 C.

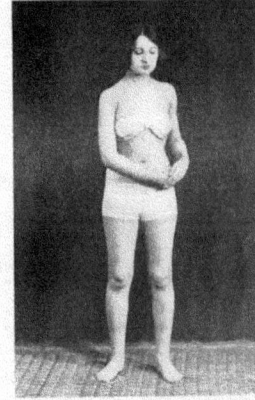

Fig. 10 D.

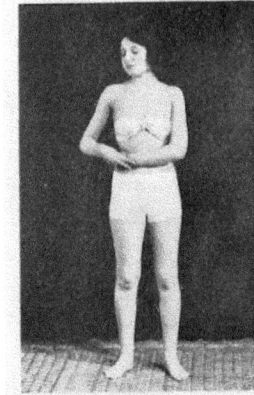

Fig. 10 E.

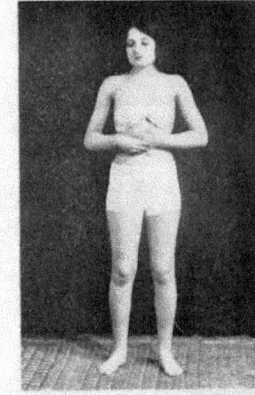

Fig. 10 F.

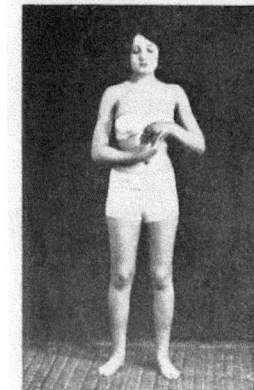

Fig. 10 G.

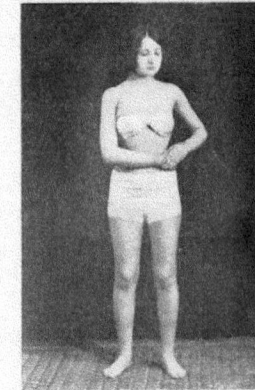

Fig. 10 H.

Fig. 10 A.   Fig. 10 B.

Fig. 10 C.   Fig. 10 D.

Fig. 10 E.   Fig. 10 F.

Fig. 10 G.   Fig. 10 H.

Place the left hand with the right on top transversely over the outer side of the right hip in such a way that the fingers of the left hand are pointing outward or around toward the back, and the hand is in line with the lower abdomen (Fig. 10 A). Stroke thus from there, straight across the lower abdomen just underneath the umbilicus to the left side, pressing continually with the right hand on top (Fig. 10 B and C).

Then stroke with the right hand and pressing with the left on top of it from the side of the left hip directly across the lower abdomen from that side, in the same way. (Fig. 10 D. Being similar to the movement just completed, only one figure is shown here.)

Now, place the left hand, with the right on top of it, again on the side of the right hip, but this time about four inches higher up, so that the thumb is just above the crest of the ilium, or hip bone (Fig. 10 E). Stroke from there, with the left hand, inward and upward underneath the border of the ribs as far as the sternum (the bone in the middle of the chest). The palm of the hand, which of course precedes the fingers, moves at first slightly transversely (Fig. 10 F). The inner side of the ends of the fingers are pressed in under the ribs with the help of the right hand until they reach the sternum or where the ribs are slanting downwards to the left side (Fig. 10 G).

Stroke now, with the right hand, the left pressing on top of it, from the side of the left hip, with the thumb just above the hip bone, inward and upward underneath the false ribs, that is, in the same way as was done with the left hand from the right side. (Fig. 10 H. Here, likewise, only one figure is shown.)

Thus, first stroke once from each opposite side across the lower abdomen, then once from each opposite side inward and upward under the ribs. The exercise has been executed once.

Five times will take about forty seconds.

NOTE I. The trunk should be kept in an upright position and not bent to the right, left or backwards. The abdominal muscles should be relaxed so that the stomach and bowels are neither distended nor contracted, but are held naturally.

NOTE II. The movements can, of course, also be done with one hand, but because pressure should be fairly strong (especially in stout people) to influence the digestive and abdominal organs and the nerve-centers properly, it is best to use both hands, one on top of the other. The strain will thus also be removed from the fingers when they are pressing inward and upward under the false ribs.

Analysis and Effects of the Combined Massage Exercise No. 10

In this exercise especial attention is given to the massaging of the internal organs, muscles, nerves and vessels of the abdomen, without any movements of the body except those of the arms.

The movements of the arms and hands in applying the massage movements, exercise the muscles of the arms, the shoulders, upper chest and back.

The massage influences the digestive organs and glands as well as all the other organs in the abdomen.

This exercise is very beneficial for all the digestive and abdominal organs in women as well as in men. (See also chapter for women, page 17, and Digestive Disorders in Supplement, page 88.)

THE COMBINED MASSAGE EXERCISE No. 11

Beating with the clenched hands (women may use the palm of the hand with the fingers outstretched), upward over each side of abdomen and chest, and bending the upper body backward at the same time; then beating similarly downward, bringing the upper body forward to an upright position, while the hands are beating downward over the chest.

Detailed Description

Position.—Standing erect, legs and feet stationary.

EXERCISE No. 11.

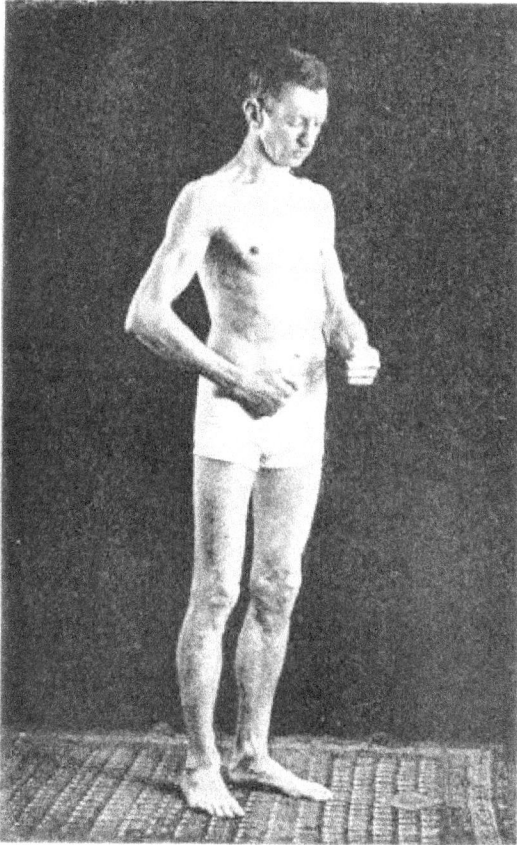 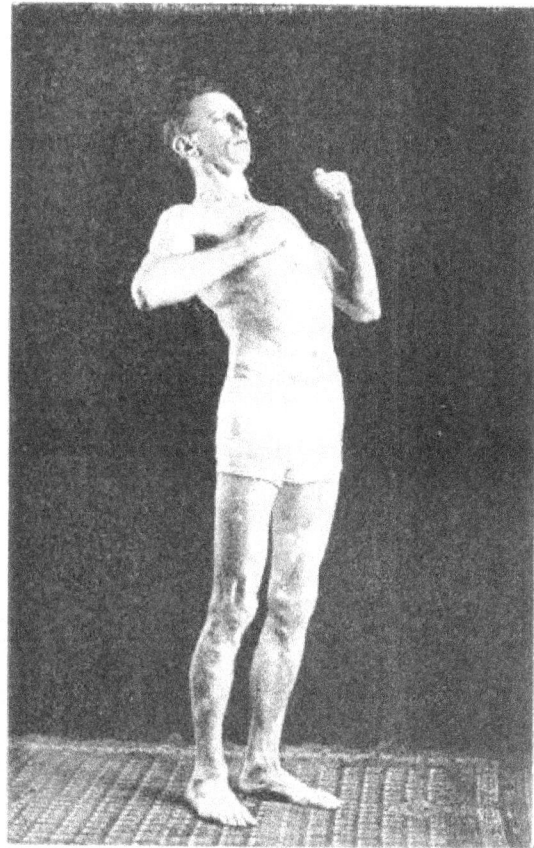

Fig. 11 A.   Fig. 11 B.

Clench the hands. With the palm and the outer side of the fingers, which are thus turned toward the body, strike first a light and quick blow with the right hand on the right side of the lower abdomen (Fig. 11 A), then similarly with the left hand on the left side of the abdomen, at the same level. Then strike with the right hand again, one or two fingers' breadth further upward on the lower right half of abdomen, and again, with the left hand, a little further up on the left side, and so forth, up over the chest. When the hands reach the lower ribs, and while they are thus beating upward, on each side of the chest, to the collar bone, the upper body is bent backward, as far as possible, but without strain (Fig. 11 B). From there, beat the same way back and downward again over chest, at the same time bringing the upper body forward to an upright position. When the hands continue down over the abdomen, the upper body is thus in a natural position.

The hands should give light, quick blows and rebound from the body each time, as in the beating of a drum.

NOTE. Women may use the palms of the hands, with the fingers outstretched and close together, when beating over the chest. Inhale the air while the upper body is being bent backward, exhale while it is brought forward to an upright position.

This exercise done five times will take about ten seconds. If counting every time when commencing to beat upward over the abdomen, it will make five counts.

Analysis and Effects of the Combined Massage Exercise No. 11

This exercise is combined in such a way that there is obtained the movements of the arms and the bending of the upper body backwards, together with the beating of the abdomen and of the chest.

The beating, which in massage is called tapotement, stimulates the nerves and contracts and stimulates the muscles, if the blows are given very lightly and quickly. Stronger and harder blows cause a benumbing effect upon the nerves, and should therefore be avoided.

The movements of the trunk and the arms and hands, in applying the beating, exercise the muscles and nerves of the arms, the shoulders, the back and the abdomen.

The beating influences the nerves, vessels, organs and muscles of the abdomen and the chest. It stimulates the heart and loosens the excretion from the lungs.

THE COMBINED MASSAGE EXERCISE No. 12

Massaging transversely over the left shoulder, continuing downward over the upper left part of the chest with the right hand, then, in the same way, over the right shoulder and upper chest with the left hand.

Detailed Description

Position.—Standing erect.

EXERCISE NO. 12.

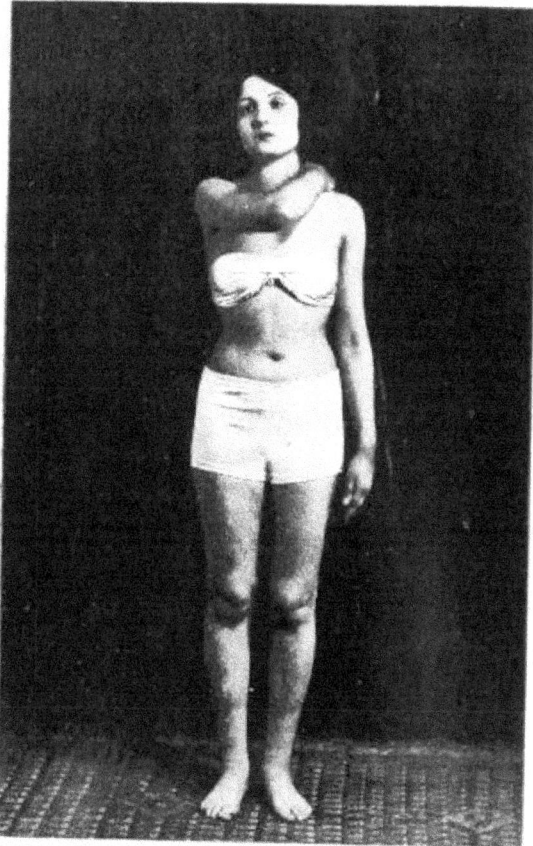 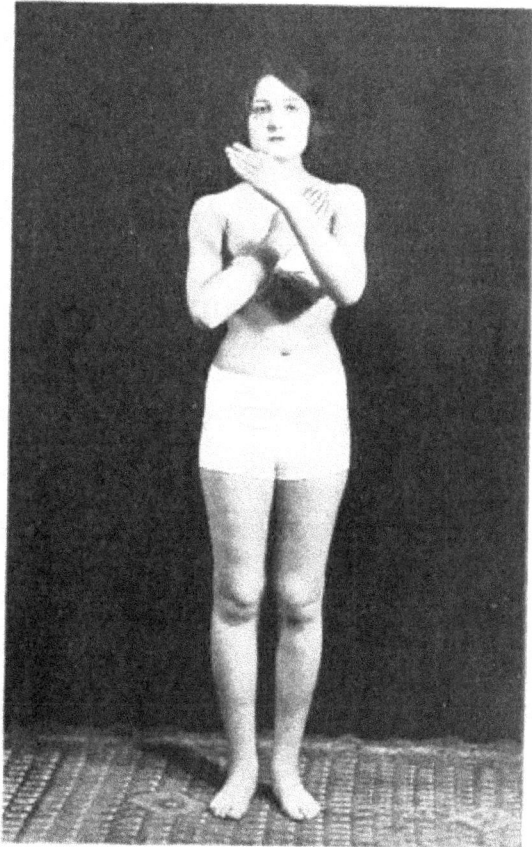

Fig. 12 A.   Fig. 12 B.

With the four fingers and thumb close, place the right hand transversely over the left shoulder in such a way that the fingers are reaching as far down on the upper back as possible, the two or three first fingers resting between the inner border of the shoulder blade and the spine, and the thumb close to the base of the neck (Fig. 12 A).

Stroke thus with the palm of the hand, the fingers pressing more or less between the shoulder blades and spine as they move upward, transversely over the shoulder, continuing down the same side of upper chest (Fig. 12 B).

While the right hand is thus stroking the left shoulder and upper chest, the left arm and hand is brought across and up over the right forearm to the right shoulder, and this shoulder is massaged continuing downward over the upper part of the left chest, in the same way, as soon as the right arm is released from the left side of chest.

The right hand is then again brought over the left shoulder and across the left forearm and that shoulder massaged, and so forth, alternately and evenly.

This exercise done five times will take about ten seconds. If counting each time when commencing to stroke each shoulder, it will be ten counts.

Note. Men may stroke downward over the chest as far as the diaphragm, if desired.

Women should only stroke as far as the breasts, and not over them.

Analysis and Effects of the Combined Massage Exercise No. 12

This exercise is combined in such a way that there is obtained the movements of the arms together with massage of the shoulders and the upper chest.

The movements of the arms and hands, in applying the massage movements, exercise the muscles and nerves of the arms, the shoulders, the upper back and the upper chest.

The massage influences the muscles, vessels and nerves of the shoulders and the upper chest. It increases the flow of blood to the muscles surrounding the lungs.

This exercise, like No. 2, is especially beneficial for stiffness in the shoulders and upper chest, resulting from golf or other over-exertion in kindred sports.

THE COMBINED MASSAGE EXERCISE No. 13

Massaging with each hand simultaneously upward over each opposite thigh, hip, lower side of body and inward and upward over nipples or breasts and upper chest and stroking down each side of the lower back and buttocks; at the same time, bending and raising the upper body.

Detailed Description

Position.—Standing erect, heels about eight inches apart, and feet nearly parallel, legs and feet kept stationary, knees straight.

Exercise No. 13.

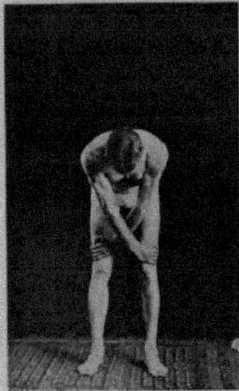
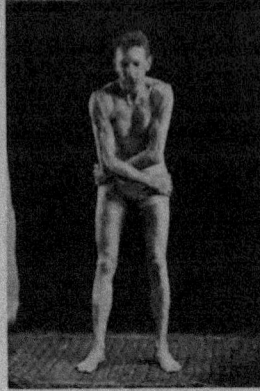

Fig. 13 A.   Fig. 13 B.

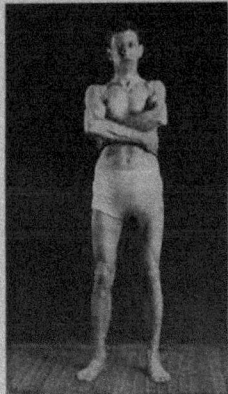
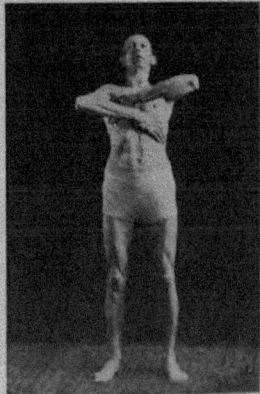

Fig. 13 C.   Fig. 13 D.

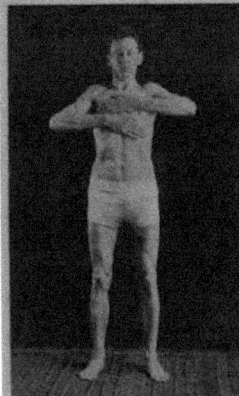
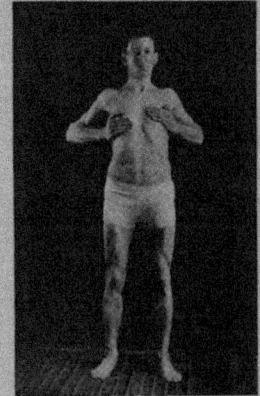

Fig. 13 E.   Fig. 13 F.

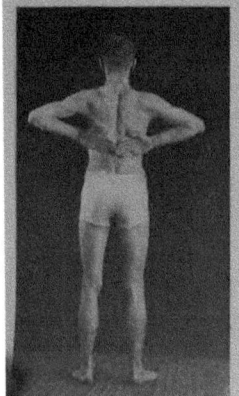
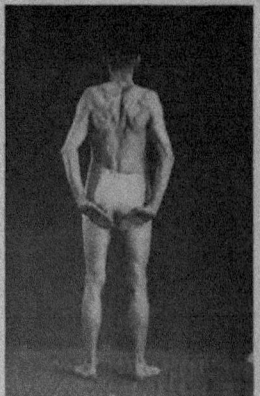

Fig. 13 G.   Fig. 13 H.

Fig. 13 A.   Fig. 13 B.

Fig. 13 C.   Fig. 13 D.

Fig. 13 E.   Fig. 13 F.

Fig. 13 G.   Fig. 13 H.

Without bending the knees, bend the upper body forward and cross the right forearm over the left, or the left over the right, placing the right hand transversely over the front of the left thigh, just above the knee; the fingers of the hand are kept close together and pointing to or around the other side of the thigh. Place the left hand in the same way and at the corresponding place on the right thigh (Fig. 13 A).

Stroke thus upward over the front of each thigh with both hands simultaneously, continuing from there, in the same way upward over hips and lower sides of the body (Fig. 13 B and C), and inward and upward over the nipples or breasts and upper chest, where the hands cross each other and continue outward to their respective sides underneath the armpits (Fig. 13 D, E and F).

Then, barely moving the arms, turn the hands from there around on each side of the back, and without here clutching the hands stroke now with the backs of the hands and fingers, downward over each side of the lower back and buttocks (Fig. 13 G and H).

The upper body is, of course, raised while the hands are stroking upward over thighs and hips and bent slightly backward while stroking inward and upward over the chest.

This exercise done five times will take about fifteen seconds.

NOTE. When stroking and pressing upward over the front part of the thigh, let the raising movement of the trunk draw the arms and hands up as far as the motion permits.

Combined with Deep Breathing

A special deep breathing exercise may be added in the following way:

Fill the lungs with air through the nose, while stroking from thighs up over sides and chest.

Retain this air in the lungs, while the hands are stroking down the back.

Exhale this air through the mouth, while bending the upper body forward in order to stroke upward over the thighs again.

Analysis and Effects of the Combined Massage Exercise No. 13

This exercise is combined in such a manner that there is obtained the movements of the arms and the bending of the trunk forward and backward, together with massage of the front of the thighs, the hips, the lower sides, the chest and breasts, the lower back and buttocks.

The movements of the body, arms and hands in applying the massage movements, exercise the muscles and nerves of the arms, the shoulders, the chest, the back, the abdomen and the hips. They also influence the abdominal organs and the heart. The nerves of the legs are stretched.

The massage influences the muscles, vessels and nerves of the front of the thighs, the hips, the lower sides, the breasts, the chest and the lower back. It also influences the heart and the kidneys.

THE COMBINED MASSAGE EXERCISE No. 14

Massaging, with the left hand, from the lower left side of the upper body and with the right hand from the upper right side of the upper body simultaneously straight across the lower and upper chest respectively to the reverse side and back again; at the same time turning the upper body to right and left.

Detailed Description

Position.—Standing erect, heels about five inches apart, feet nearly parallel, legs and feet stationary.

EXERCISE NO. 14.

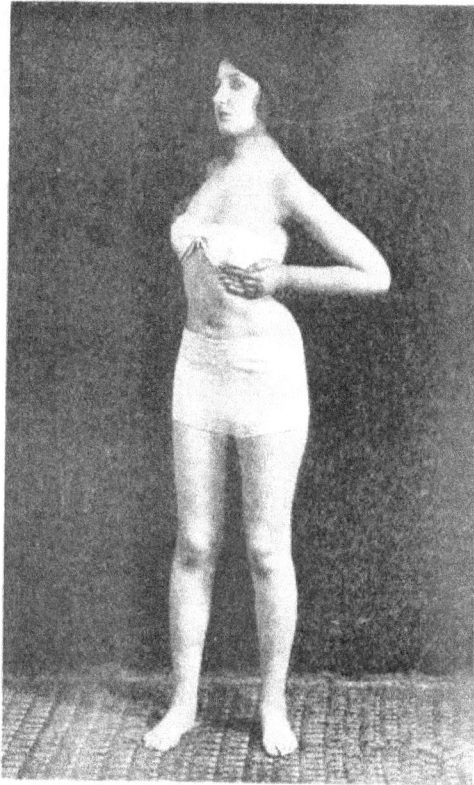

Fig. 14 A.

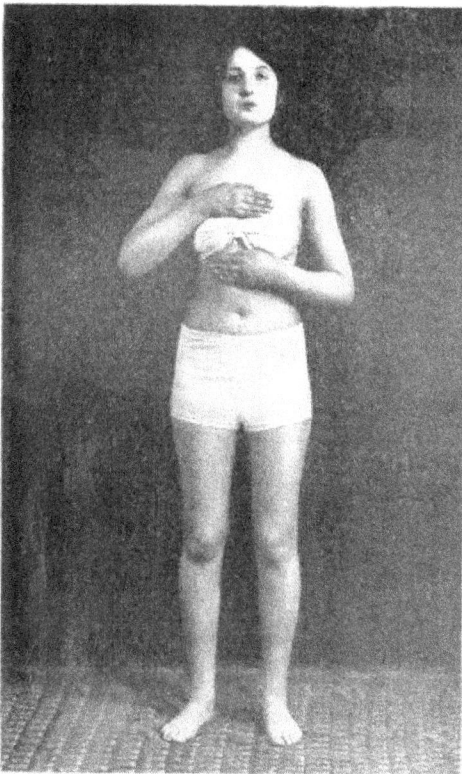

Fig. 14 B.

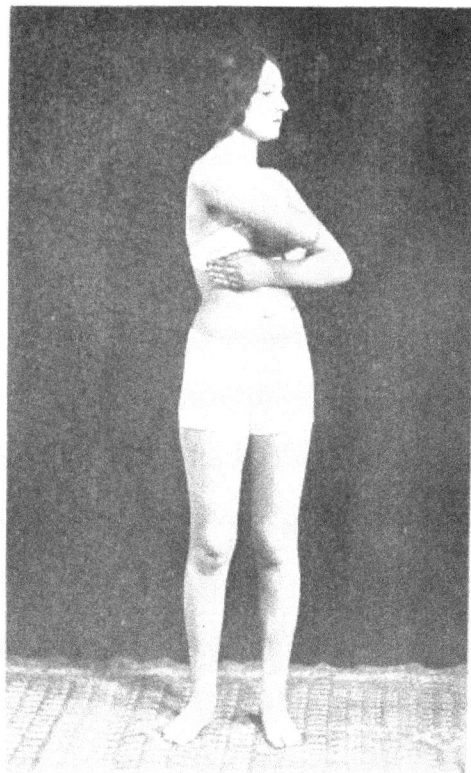

Fig. 14 C.

Fig. 14 A.

Fig. 14 B.   Fig. 14 C.

Place the left hand, with the four fingers and thumb close, transversely on the lower left side of the body, underneath the line of the nipple or breast, and in such a way that the fingers are pointing toward the middle of the chest. Place the right hand in the same way on the upper right side of the body, just underneath the armpits (Fig. 14 A).

Now, stroke with both hands, from each side at the same time, directly across the chest and as far over on the opposite side as possible (Fig. 14 B and C). Stroke back again the same way.

The left hand thus strokes from the left side underneath the nipples or breasts over on the right side and back again, while the right hand strokes from the right side across the upper chest, over on the left side and back again.

At the same time, turn the upper body slowly from side to side without altering the position of the legs and feet. The turning of the body and the stroking should be done evenly and not jerkingly.

This exercise done five times will take about fifteen seconds. If counting each time the trunk is turned to either side, it will be ten counts.

Exercise No. 14 A

(*Combined with Rolling of the Trunk*)

The massaging over the chest as done in No. 14 may also be done, while the trunk is rolled around in the following way:

Place the feet further away from each other—about ten inches.

Begin stroking the chest, as described. Without altering the position of the legs and feet, bend the upper body forward; from there roll and bend it over to the right, continuing rolling and bending it backward, then to the left and around to the front, terminating in a forward bending. Stop here and with the body still bent, roll in opposite direction, that is, to the left, back, right and front.

The hands are, of course, stroking evenly across the chest during the rolling.

The trunk may be rolled around first two or three times to the right, and then two or three times to the left.

Three times each way around is equivalent to five executions.

This exercise done five times will take about twenty seconds.

Analysis and Effects of the Combined Massage Exercise No. 14

This exercise is combined in such a way that there is obtained the movements of the arms and the turning of the trunk, together with the massage of the chest and the upper sides of the body.

The movements of the body and arms and hands in applying the massage movements, exercise the muscles and nerves of the arms, the shoulders, the upper and lower back, the sides and the abdomen. This also influences the kidneys.

The massage influences the muscles and nerves of the chest and the sides, likewise, the heart, the liver and lungs.

Effects of Exercise No. 14 A

In No. 14 A the rolling exercises the muscles and nerves of the abdomen and lower sides to a greater extent than does the turning in exercise No. 14.

PROPER BREATHING

Nothing is more important than breathing for maintaining life, and it should be given much more attention than is customary. This may be done not only by practicing the special and general breathing exercises for several minutes one or several times daily, but also by acquiring the habit of proper breathing all the time. It is a curious fact that when the stomach is in need of more food, it is filled and sometimes to excess, but although the lungs are always in need of more air, they are mostly only filled about one-half and not completely, and this in spite of the fact that air is one of the few gifts of life.

In order that the reader may notice the effect of proper natural breathing and to acquire the habit, it may be advisable to try the following experiment:

Place a watch nearby. Breathe slowly, deeply and regularly for one or several minutes, inhaling the air each time through the nose and exhaling it either the same way or through both nose and mouth simultaneously. From twelve to sixteen respirations should be done per minute.

Try occasionally to breathe with the diaphragm, that is, instead of first allowing the chest to expand, when inhaling, push the abdomen and diaphragm out first during the beginning of the inhalation and the chest during the latter half part of it. This is beneficial for all the digestive organs and their nerves. The most important thing is to breathe deeply, so that the air also reaches the bottom or points of the lungs. Of course, twelve or sixteen respirations can be taken per minute and the lungs become only half-filled just the same. This will not be of any benefit. On the contrary, it might cause anaemia, and its accompanists, such as neurasthenia, melancholia, fear, etc. Breathing in the right way will produce better blood, more nerve power, and last, but not least, a good humor.

Apropos humor,—there are authors who, now and then in the titles of their books or articles, admonish one to be cheerful, to laugh and smile so as to avoid illness. Further perusal of the text, however, will show that they admit that this depends chiefly upon the physical condition, and they advise the practice of exercises, in order to make people physically fit first. This is, of course, true, since it is difficult for most people to be of a good disposition and smile and laugh when the body is not in fit condition.

SPECIAL AND GENERAL DEEP BREATHING EXERCISES

These breathing exercises done separately or between the massage exercises will develop the chest and lungs. Causing more oxygen to be introduced into the blood and increased elimination of carbonic-acid gas, the blood is enriched, the energy increased and power developed to withstand or repulse attacks of disease. A direct as well as an indirect influence is also produced upon all the vital organs of the body.

The Special Deep Breathing Exercise
No. I

Position.—Standing or sitting erect, with shoulders back, but without strain, arms hung loosely downward to sides.

1. Inhale as deeply as possible through the nose.

2. Retain the air for one or two seconds.

3. Join the lips in such a way that a small opening remains in the middle and throw only a small quantity of air violently through this opening; retain the respiration, again throw out a little air in the same way; retain again, and so forth, in the same way, until the lungs are completely emptied of air.

4. Take a shorter but deep breath, lasting from three to five seconds.

This exercise acts as a washer and cleanser of the lungs in forcing the pure air into the corners of the lungs and pushing out the foul air accumulated.

The Special Deep Breathing Exercise
No. II

Position.—Standing or sitting erect, with shoulders back, but without strain, arms hung loosely downward to sides.

1. Inhale as deeply as possible.

2. Retain the air in the lungs as long as possible, without strain.

3. Exhale the air vigorously through the open mouth.

This exercise has a beneficial influence upon the system of respiration, the blood and the nervous system.

The Special Deep Breathing Exercise
No. III

Position.—Standing erect, with shoulders back, but without strain, arms hung loosely downward to sides.

1. Inhale as deeply as possible through the nose.

2. Stretch both arms easily outward to sides in line with shoulders.

3. Bring the hands to the shoulders, gradually contracting the hands in such a way that when they reach the shoulders the fists are very strongly clenched.

4. During this tension of the muscles, bend the fists rapidly outward and inward from ten to twenty times.

5. Exhale the air vigorously through the mouth, at the same time dropping the arms loosely downward to sides.

6. Take a shorter but deep breath, lasting three to five seconds.

Besides being beneficial to the lungs, the respiratory muscles and the heart; this exercise is also very beneficial for the vitality of the nerves, especially those of the brachial plexus (the nerves of the arms, shoulders, upper back and upper chest).

The General Deep Breathing Exercise
A

1. Arms hanging loosely at sides or place hands on hips, elbows and shoulders thrown backward, without strain.

2. Inhale as deeply as possible, at the same time rising on toes.

3. Exhale through the mouth, at the same time sinking on heels.

The General Deep Breathing Exercise
B

Position.—Arms outstretched horizontally to the front and parallel to each other.

1. Inhale as deeply as possible, at the same time bringing the arms horizontally outward to the sides and continuing as far back as possible, while rising on toes.

2. Exhale through the mouth while dropping the arms slowly downward to the sides and sinking on heels.

Exercises *A* and *B* may also be done without rising on toes, but this exercise greatly strengthens the feet and ankles and the muscles of the legs and gives a good poise.

When practicing the breathing exercises *A* and *B*, both legs may be bent and stretched at the same time, and this will further strengthen the legs.

All these breathing exercises are especially beneficial for singers and public speakers.

SPECIAL REMARKS

Always inhale through the nose.

The breathing exercises may, of course, be practiced separately either indoors or outdoors.

If practiced indoors, it is important to have good ventilation in the room.

If slight dizziness should result when practicing the special breathing exercises separately, begin moderately, and as the lungs become stronger, this feeling will gradually diminish.

Practicing the three special deep breathing exercises five times each, without any long pause between, should consume about five minutes. From five to ten minutes is sufficient for one performance and, as a rule, this time limit should not be exceeded. They can, of course, be practiced several times a day.

SYNOPTIC REVIEW OF THE COMBINED MASSAGE EXERCISES

This is added to assist ready memorization of the exercises and their order, after having studied and learned them from the detailed description.

In the margin is stated the average time—in seconds—for doing each massage exercise five times and likewise the time limit—also in seconds—for interval breathing where indicated.

It will thus serve as a guide when practicing all the exercises together as a daily course.

No. 1

TEMPLE, HEAD, NECK AND THROAT

Massaging (stroking and pressing) the temple, head, neck and throat; at the same time bending the head forward and backward.

30 sec.

At this and at the other intervals where it is indicated, practice the special deep breathing exercise No. 1, once. Or

Practice the general deep breathing exercise A once or twice, but without rising on toes. Time not to exceed fifteen seconds.

15 sec.

If special deep breathing is done while practicing the massage exercises themselves, no deep breathing should be done between them.

No. 2

ARMS, SIDES AND ACROSS LOWER CHEST

Massaging (stroking and pressing) each arm, side and directly across the lower chest alternately; and at the same time exercising the arms and shoulders.	**30 sec.**
Deep Breathing	**15 sec.**

No. 3 or (3 A—from a lying position)

EACH LEG AND STRAIGHT ACROSS ABDOMEN, ALTERNATELY

(Similar to Rowing)

Massaging (stroking and pressing) with both hands, first the right leg, from ankle upward, and straight across abdomen to the left side, then the left leg and straight across abdomen to the right side; at the same time bending and stretching the legs and also bending and raising the trunk.	**30 sec.**
Deep Breathing	**15 sec.**

No. 4

EACH SIDE OF BODY AND STRAIGHT ACROSS LOWER CHEST, ALTERNATELY

Massaging (stroking and pressing) each side of body, from side of thigh, at knee upward and straight across the lower chest, alternately, with each hand; at the same time bending the trunk from side to side.	**15 sec.**
Deep Breathing	**15 sec.**

No. 5

BOTH LEGS, ACROSS LOWER CHEST AND ABDOMEN INWARD AND UPWARD ACROSS CHEST, OUTWARD TO ARMPITS AND DOWN THE BACK AND BUTTOCKS

Massaging (stroking and pressing) each leg from	**30 sec.**

behind, simultaneously with each hand, upward over each hip, straight across the lower chest (from the left side with the left hand) and at the same time straight across the abdomen (from the right side with the right hand) to opposite sides, from there inward and upward across chest, outward to armpits, then downward on each side of lower back and buttocks; at the same time bending and raising the trunk.

<table>
<tr><td>Deep Breathing</td><td>**15 sec.**</td></tr>
</table>

No. 6

BOTH SIDES OF BACK AND BUTTOCKS—TURNING

Massaging (stroking and pressing) each side of lower back and buttocks, simultaneously with each hand; at the same time turning the trunk to the right and left.

10 sec.

<table>
<tr><td>Deep Breathing</td><td>**15 sec.**</td></tr>
</table>

No. 7

Massaging (stroking and pressing) the right leg and straight across abdomen, as in exercise No. 3; then the right arm, down the right side and across lower chest, as in exercise No. 2; then the left leg and across abdomen; and the left arm, side and across lower chest; then from each opposite side simultaneously, inward and upward across chest, outward to armpits; then downward on each side of the back and buttocks; finally swinging the arms around to the front and vibrating or pushing the skin and underlying tissues sideways on each opposite side of lower chest; at the same time bending and stretching the legs more or less, and also bending and raising the trunk.

60 sec.

Deep Breathing   **15 sec.**

No. 8

EACH SIDE OF LOWER BACK—TURNING

Massaging (stroking and pressing) down each side
of lower back alternately with each hand; at the same   **20 sec.**
time turning the trunk to the right and left.

Deep Breathing   **15 sec.**

No. 9 or (9 A with additional arm movement)

EACH OUTER SIDE OF OPPOSITE THIGH, OPPOSITE HIP, INWARD
AND UPWARD ACROSS CHEST, OUTWARD TO ARMPIT,
ALTERNATELY

Massaging (stroking and pressing) from each outer
side of opposite thigh, upward over opposite hip and
inward and upward across chest, outward to armpit,
alternately with each hand; at the same time turning
and bending the trunk slightly forward and also   **25 sec.**
bending it from side to side. (If the exercise is done ten
times or more, practice both No. 9 and 9 A, half the
number of times each.)

Deep Breathing   **15 sec.**

No. 10

ABDOMEN

Massaging (stroking and pressing) with the left hand   **40 sec.**
from the side of the right hip, straight across the lower
abdomen; then the same movement with the right
hand, from the left side; thereafter, again with the left
hand, from the right hip, inward and upward
underneath the false ribs to the end of the breast bone;

then the same movement, with the right hand, from the left side,—the other hand pressing on top of the one which is massaging.

Deep Breathing   **15 sec.**

No. 11

BEATING OVER ABDOMEN AND CHEST

Beating upward over abdomen and chest and down; at the same time bending the trunk backward and forward to upright position.   **10 sec.**

Deep Breathing   **15 sec.**

No. 2—Repeated

ARMS ONLY

Practice here again Massage Exercise No. 2, but without massaging down sides and across lower chest —five times will here be sufficient.   **30 sec.**

No Deep Breathing Here

No. 12

SHOULDERS AND UPPER CHEST

Massaging (stroking and pressing) transversely over the left shoulder, downward over the upper left chest with the right hand; then across the right shoulder and downward over the upper right chest, in the same way, with the left hand, and so forth, alternately.   **10 sec.**

Deep Breathing   **15 sec.**

No. 13

BOTH FRONT ASPECTS OF OPPOSITE THIGHS, HIPS AND SIDES
OF LOWER BODY, INWARD AND UPWARD ACROSS CHEST AND
DOWNWARD ON BACK AND BUTTOCKS

Massaging (stroking and pressing) each upper leg in front simultaneously, from just above the knees, upwards over hips and lower sides of body, with arms crossed (the right leg, hip and lower side with the left hand, and the left leg, hip and lower side with the right), continuing inward and upward across chest, outward to armpits, and downward over each side of lower back and buttocks; at the same time bending the trunk forward and backward.   **15 sec.**

Deep Breathing   **15 sec.**

No. 14

UPPER AND LOWER CHEST—TURNING

Massaging (stroking and pressing) from the lower right side of the upper body with the right hand, and from the upper left side of the upper body with the left hand simultaneously straight across the lower and upper chest to opposite sides and back again; at the same time turning the trunk to the right and left.   **15 sec.**

No Deep Breathing at this Interval

No. 14 A

Massaging (stroking and pressing) straight across the upper and lower chest, as in exercise No. 14, but instead of turning, roll the trunk around in a circle.   **20 sec.**

Three times each way around is equivalent to five executions.

Deep Breathing	15 sec.
Total	**10 minutes**

(Without considering the pauses between the massage exercises and the deep breathing exercises.)

Practicing thus all the combined massage exercises five times each, and using fifteen seconds for the deep breathing at each of those intervals, where indicated, will require about twelve minutes, provided, of course, that the pauses between the massage exercises and the deep breathing exercises are not too long.

The five-times-limit is purely arbitrary and has been selected merely as an illustration.

Practicing all the massage exercises ten times each, and in the manner just explained, will not necessarily make the whole performance last twice as long, as when they are practiced five times each, because the time for the breathing exercises will remain the same.

When explaining in the detailed description how special deep breathing can be done during the practice of massage exercises Nos. 5, 7 and 13, it was with the particular intention that this should be done chiefly in instances where one or two of these exercises are practiced separately and when the performer has only a few minutes to spare. However, even when all the massage exercises are practiced together, Nos. 5, 7 and 13 may also be performed in that way, but in that case only natural breathing and no special deep breathing exercises should be done at the intervals.

On the whole, practice of a deep breathing exercise at the intervals is more practical, although the one method is about as beneficial as the other. But to do special deep breathing during the practice of some of the exercises themselves, as well as at the intervals in the same performance would be out of proportion.

HOW THE NUMBER OF EXERCISES FOR ONE PERFORMANCE CAN BEST BE DECREASED

Elderly people, children and others whose memory is not of the best and who may, therefore, find it inconvenient to remember all the exercises in the beginning or later can shorten the number of exercises for one performance in the following ways:

Eleven Massage Exercises
Nos. 1, 2, 3, 4, 5, 9, 10, 12, 13, 14 and 14 A

Nine Massage Exercises
Nos. 1, 2, 3, 4, 5, 10, 12, 13 and 14

Seven Massage Exercises
Nos. 1, 2, 3, 4, 5, 13 and 14

Six Massage Exercises
Nos. 1, 2, 3, 5, 9 and 14

Five Massage Exercises
Nos. 1, 4, 7, 13 and 14

Of course, these groupings may be modified in any other order and number with benefit, but the ones here indicated are the best and most practical. The ideal manner, however, is to practice all the exercises together in the order mentioned.

ANOTHER SYSTEM
PRACTICING THE MOVEMENTS OF THE BODY WITHOUT THE MASSAGE

The movements or exercises of the arms, legs and the body in the combined massage exercises may also be done without the massage.

Thus, when dressed, the arms, legs and trunk may perform the same movements as when massaging, but without the hands touching the clothes. Done in this way, the hands should move at a distance of about two inches from the clothes and be firmly clenched while exercising, thus contracting and concentrating on the muscles of the arms and also as far as possible concentrating the mind on those other parts of the body put into play by an exercise.

In this way another concentration system, similar if not better than the Indian exercises, is obtained. Of course, this is not nearly as efficient as when done without clothes and with the addition of the massage. It might be desirable to try them in that way at a time when exercise is needed, and there is no time, or convenience for the removal of clothes.

Deep breathing can also with great benefit be combined to some of these exercises in the same way as explained under the detailed description of the massage exercises.

SUPPLEMENT
HOW THE EXERCISES MAY BE UTILIZED IN SOME DISEASED AND DISORDERED CONDITIONS OF THE BODY

The massage exercises and deep breathing exercises may be used with benefit in certain stages of different diseases. This should, of course, be done only on the recommendation of a physician.

Inasmuch as the same disease does not attack all people to the same degree, it is, of course, impossible to state exactly when or at which stage of a disease the patient might begin to practice the exercises. Neither can it be said precisely how long an exercise or performance shall last in each case; it will vary from five to twenty minutes. This is a matter for the family physician to decide; however, the following hints may be in order. If the use of the exercises practiced moderately is recommended, begin them slowly for five or ten minutes daily (or as long as advised by the doctor) with a light pressure of the hands, and continue thus for several days. The exercises can then be made more vigorous by increasing the pressure of the hands to a moderate or stronger degree. The time can then likewise be increased to fifteen or twenty minutes in proportion to the improvement in the condition and strength of the performer.

It is not meant to imply that it is necessary to immediately hurry to a doctor or hospital when disorders of a mild character occur; for instance, a slight pain or stiffness in the muscles of one of the limbs or other part of the body, a headache, obesity without complications or slight constipation.

If three or more massage exercises are recommended for one performance, a general deep breathing exercise can likewise be practiced between each of those.

Here may be noted, especially for the interest of physicians, the particular exercises which are most suitable for use in various diseases. There are other conditions than the ones mentioned below, in which the exercises might be used with benefit, but the following are the most important:

Anaemia

Headache

Disorders of the Digestive System

Disorders of the Liver

Diabetes

Affections of the Lungs

Disordered Conditions of the Heart

Insomnia

Muscular Disorders

Nervous Diseases

Obesity

Curvature of the Spine

ANAEMIA

All the massage exercises may be practiced once or twice daily. In addition, all the deep breathing exercises may be done separately, without strain, for five or ten minutes, twice daily.

HEADACHE

Here special reference is made to massage exercise No. 1, although all the exercises will prove of indirect benefit.

DISORDERS OF THE DIGESTIVE SYSTEM

(Constipation—Gas in the Stomach—Stasis—Dilatation of the Stomach—Chronic Dyspepsia—Deficient Peristaltic Action, etc.)

Reference is here made especially to massage exercise No. 10, and also to Nos. 3 and 5. All the deep breathing exercises may be used. If the patient is so weak that the trunk cannot be bent much, No. 10 may be practiced first and Nos. 3 and 5 later. No. 10 can even be practiced by patients confined to bed.

For dilatation of the stomach, chronic dyspepsia and conditions of stasis, No. 10 is very beneficial, and may be used for ten or fifteen minutes two or three times a day. It causes contraction of the stomach, the pylorus is opened and the contents are emptied into the duodenum. Sour and burning eructations, bad breath and taste in the mouth will disappear. In these cases it is best to practice the exercise from four to five hours after a meal. (The massage movements in No. 10 has been taught by the author to several mothers from out of town, who have applied them with success to their babies suffering from gas in the stomach and indigestion caused by nervous disorders.)

In order to increase the flow of bile, pancreatic juice and the succus entericus and to get a mixture of these, a well-known medical authority in Europe massaged (stroking and pressing) the abdomen from the right side toward the median line for about half an hour after the stomach digestion had ceased. The average amount of the juices thus obtained in each of twenty cases was from 40 to 50 c.c. This movement is included in massage exercise No. 10 and also somewhat in exercises Nos. 3 and 5.

In a case of a dropped stomach or colon, a special movement of stroking and pressing (especially with the fingers) may be used across the abdomen in an upward direction, from each opposite side of the lower abdomen, thus crossing the abdomen with each hand, alternately.

A good movement for breaking up adhesions in the region of the appendix is stroking with the fingers of the right hand (pressing on top with the left) upward over the appendix, the ascending colon and then continuing over the transverse colon. For adhesions in the left side of the abdomen a similar movement with the fingers of the left hand is recommended. Massage exercises Nos. 10 and 3 are also here beneficial.

In order to relieve the bowels of their distension, one doctor in New York advocated massaging the abdomen thirty hours after operations for appendicitis and hernia.

DISORDERS OF THE LIVER

Reference is here made to massage exercises Nos. 2, 3, 4, 6, 8, 14 and 14 A, as well as to all the deep breathing exercises.

They will stimulate the secretion of the bile from the blood and cause readier transformation of excess sugar into glycogen.

The massage exercises are also beneficial for hepatic engorgement.

DIABETES

All the massage and deep breathing exercises are recommended for the reason that they cause an increased oxygenation in all parts of the body and will therefore help to prevent abnormal deposits of sugar.

AFFECTIONS OF THE LUNGS

(Pneumonia—Tuberculosis—Asthma)

Massage exercises Nos. 2 and 14 are here especially referred to as well as all the deep breathing exercises.

Convalescence from pneumonia has been shortened and eased by massaging the painful muscles which are at times concomitants of lung affections.

The massaging over the chest will cause freer breathing and expectoration.

In the first stage of tuberculosis all the massage exercises done with a light or moderate pressure and all the deep breathing exercises, practiced once or twice daily are beneficial.

In asthma all the exercises are likewise recommended.

DISORDERED CONDITIONS OF THE HEART

In severe cases, massage exercises Nos. 2 and 14 may be used, with a light pressure for five minutes, two or three times a day. The special deep breathing exercise No. 2 and the general deep breathing exercises may also be practiced slowly and without strain.

For milder cases reference is made to massage exercises Nos. 2, 4, 5, 9, 13 and 14.

INSOMNIA

All the massage exercises practiced for ten or fifteen minutes without exertion half an hour before going to bed are recommended.

MUSCULAR DISORDERS

(Stiffness and Pain—Atrophy and Distrophy—Lumbago)

For stiffness in the neck, use massage exercise No. 1.

For stiffness in the shoulders, massage exercise No. 12 is beneficial.

For muscular disturbance in an arm, massage exercise No. 2 is recommended.

For pain in the muscles of the lower back, massage exercises Nos. 6 and 8 are very beneficial.

For muscular disturbance in the lower limbs, massage exercises Nos. 3 and 3 A may be used.

For stiffness in the muscles of the upper chest, massage exercises Nos. 12 and 14 are indicated.

NERVOUS DISEASES

(Neuritis—Neuralgia—Sciatica—General Nervousness or Neurasthenia)

In any kind of nervous disease of a mild character, all the massage exercises and the deep breathing exercises might be practiced two or three times a day.

For neuritis or neuralgia in the arms, massage exercise No. 2 can be practiced, after the acute stage has passed.

For facial neuralgia, massage exercise No. 1 is recommended, with stroking from each cheek instead of from the temple.

In sciatica, massage exercise No. 3 is beneficial; if the attack is severe exercise No. 3 A may be used.

In cases of general nervousness or debility resulting from overwork, strain or other cause, all the massage exercises can be used from ten to twenty minutes two or three times a day, according to the condition of the patient.

In cases of partial paralysis of an arm or leg, exercises Nos. 2, 3 or 3 A may be used respectively.

OBESITY

All the massage and deep breathing exercises are recommended.

If most pronounced, about the waist, reference is especially made to massage exercises Nos. 3, 3 A, 5, 7, 10, 11 and 14 A.

In the case that the heart and other organs are not especially affected, the performer may practice these massage exercises with a strong pressure for twenty minutes or more, or until practically tired out.

CURVATURE OF THE SPINE

Although all the massage exercises may here be used with benefit, Nos. 6, 8, 13, 5 and 1 are especially referred to.

In hospitals where children (mostly girls from ten to sixteen years of age) attend gymnastic classes for correction of the spine no massage treatment is given them as a rule. This is probably because there is no time for both exercises and massage treatment. The latter, however, would greatly help to nourish and strengthen the weak muscles which are associated with curvatures of the spine.

In massage exercises Nos. 6 and 8, and to a lesser degree in Nos. 13 and 5, massage of each side of the back (except the uppermost parts) is obtained at the same time. No. 1 is included in the ones especially recommended, because the movements of the arms in this exercise strengthens the upper part of the back.

In all diseased or disordered conditions, proper breathing at all times should be remembered.